Reproductive Ethics in Clinical Practice

Reproductive Ethics in Clinical Practice

Preventing, Initiating, and Managing Pregnancy and Delivery

Essays Inspired by the MacLean Center for Clinical Medical Ethics Lecture Series

Edited by

JULIE CHOR, MD, MPH

*Assistant Professor, Obstetrics and Gynecology,
Pritzker School of Medicine, The University of Chicago*

*Assistant Director, MacLean Center for Clinical Medical Ethics,
The University of Chicago*

KATIE WATSON, JD

*Associate Professor, Medical Social Sciences, Medical Education,
and Obstetrics and Gynecology, Feinberg School of Medicine,
Northwestern University*

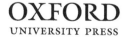

OXFORD
UNIVERSITY PRESS

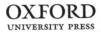

Oxford University Press is a department of the University of Oxford. It furthers
the University's objective of excellence in research, scholarship, and education
by publishing worldwide. Oxford is a registered trade mark of Oxford University
Press in the UK and certain other countries.

Published in the United States of America by Oxford University Press
198 Madison Avenue, New York, NY 10016, United States of America.

Library of Congress Cataloging-in-Publication Data
Names: Chor, Julie, editor. | Watson, Katie, editor.
Title: Reproductive ethics in clinical practice / editors, Julie Chor,
Katie Watson.
Description: New York, NY : Oxford University Press, [2021] | Includes
bibliographical references and index.
Identifiers: LCCN 2021008369 (print) | LCCN 2021008370 (ebook) | ISBN
9780190873028 (hardback) | ISBN 9780190873011 (paperback) | ISBN
9780190873059 (epub) | ISBN 9780190873035
Subjects: MESH: Reproductive Medicine—ethics | Essay
Classification: LCC RG133.5 (print) | LCC RG133.5 (ebook) | NLM WQ 9 |
DDC 176/.2—dc23
LC record available at https://lccn.loc.gov/2021008369

DOI: 10.1093/med/9780190873028.001.0001

This material is not intended to be, and should not be considered, a substitute for medical or other professional
advice. Treatment for the conditions described in this material is highly dependent on the individual circumstances.
And, while this material is designed to offer accurate information with respect to the subject matter covered and
to be current as of the time it was written, research and knowledge about medical and health issues is constantly
evolving and dose schedules for medications are being revised continually, with new side effects recognized and
accounted for regularly. Readers must therefore always check the product information and clinical procedures
with the most up-to-date published product information and data sheets provided by the manufacturers and the
most recent codes of conduct and safety regulation. The publisher and the authors make no representations or
warranties to readers, express or implied, as to the accuracy or completeness of this material. Without limiting the
foregoing, the publisher and the authors make no representations or warranties as to the accuracy or efficacy of
the drug dosages mentioned in the material. The authors and the publisher do not accept, and expressly disclaim,
any responsibility for any liability, loss, or risk that may be claimed or incurred as a consequence of the use and/or
application of any of the contents of this material.

Hardback printed by Bridgeport National Bindery, Inc., United States of America

Deepest gratitude to the Charlie Boys for their constant love and support.
—JC

For my grandmothers, both nurses, for modeling women at work and caring for others as a profession.
—KW

Contents

Acknowledgments

Julie Chor and Katie Watson thank the MacLean Center for Clinical Medical Ethics at the University of Chicago and Dr. Mark Siegler, Director of the MacLean Center, for their support of the production of this book, for the year-long lecture series that served as the foundation for this volume, and for the Fellowship training that first taught us to think deeply about the ethical complexity and impact of patient–healthcare professional interactions.

About the Authors

Stephen D. Brown, MD, is a pediatric radiologist at Boston Children's Hospital and immediate past Director of the Hospital's Institute for Professionalism and Ethical Practice. He is Associate Professor of Radiology at Harvard Medical School, where he serves on the core faculty in the medical student Medical Ethics and Professionalism curriculum and as a Capstone Seminar faculty member in the MBE program. Dr. Brown attended the University of Pennsylvania School of Medicine, completed a diagnostic radiology residency at Massachusetts General Hospital, and fellowships in pediatric radiology and pediatric interventional radiology at Boston Children's Hospital. He also completed the 2003–2004 Harvard Medical School Fellowship in Bioethics, where the ideas for his book chapter were conceived, with empirical work subsequently funded through a Boston Children's Hospital Faculty Career Development Award, the American Roentgen Ray Society Leonard Berlin Scholarship in Medical Professionalism, and grants from the Kornfeld Program in Bioethics and Patient Care, the Greenwall Foundation, and the Harvard University Milton Fund.

Laurence Brunet, MLS, is a legal scholar and research associate of the Institut des sciences juridique et philosophique de la Sorbonne (UMR 8103) at the Université de Paris I. While lecturing on Fundamental Rights and Personal Law at the Institut d'Etudes Judiciaires of the Université de Paris XI, she also is a legal counsel at the Centre de Référence des Maladies Rares du Développement Génital (DEVGEN) of the Kremlin Bicêtre Hospital. Her research focuses on the interactions between family law and advances in scientific and medical research, with special emphasis on new family configurations, children born of surrogacy, and the status of transgender individuals.

Frank A. Chervenak, MD, MMM, is Professor and Chair of Obstetrics and Gynecology, Lenox Hill Hospital and Chair and Associate Dean for International Medicine at the Zucker School of Medicine at Hofstra/Northwell in New York. He is a member of the US National Academy of

Medicine and has received honorary doctorates at 11 medical universities throughout the world. He has collaborated for 38 years with Dr. Laurence B. McCullough on ethics in obstetrics and gynecology, resulting in 286 peer-reviewed papers and three books. The most recent of these, co-authored with Dr. John H. Coverdale (Professor of Psychiatry and Medical Ethics, Baylor College of Medicine), *Professional Ethics in Obstetrics and Gynecology*, was published by Cambridge University Press in 2020.

Julie Chor, MD, MPH, is an Assistant Professor of Obstetrics and Gynecology and an Assistant Director of the MacLean Center for Clinical Medical Ethics at the University of Chicago. After completing medical school at the University of Chicago's Pritzker School of Medicine, Dr. Chor completed her Obstetrics and Gynecology residency, Fellowship in Complex Family Planning, and MPH at the University of Illinois at Chicago. Her academic and clinical work focus on understanding and addressing barriers that adolescents and young adults face in seeking and obtaining reproductive health care. Dr. Chor also serves as a member of the American College of Obstetricians and Gynecologists' Committee on Ethics.

Bruno Ramalho de Carvalho, MD, MSc, MBA, is a board-certified specialist in gynecology and human assisted reproduction. After completing medical school at the Federal University of Uberlândia, Minas Gerais, Brazil, Dr. Bruno completed his obstetrics and gynecology, and assisted reproduction residency and MSc at the University of São Paulo in Ribeirão Preto, São Paulo, Brazil. His work focuses on providing reproductive health assistance, with special interest on fertility preservation, either for medical or social reasons. He also serves as a member of the Brazilian Federation of Gynecology and Obstetrics Associations' National Specialty Commission on Human Reproduction and as a member of the clinical staff of Hospital Sírio-Libanês in Brasília, Federal District, Brazil.

Jeanne Flavin, PhD, is Professor of Sociology at Fordham University in New York City. She received a 2013 Sociologists for Women in Society award for social action and a 2009 Fulbright research award to study women, family, and crime in South Africa. Her publications include the award-winning *Our Bodies, Our Crimes: Policing Women's Reproduction in America* (New York University Press, 2009) and the co-edited volume, *Race, Gender, and Punishment: From Colonialism to the War on Terror* (Rutgers University

Press, 2007). Her current research, undertaken in partnership with National Advocates for Pregnant Women, documents the assaults on the personhood of pregnant people, including women whose poverty, race, and/or mental health make them vulnerable targets for arrest and prosecution on the basis of their actions or inactions during pregnancy, and other abuses of state power.

Véronique Fournier, MD, PhD, founded the first clinical ethics service support in France in 2002 and directed it for 18 years. She conceived this service after having been delegated by the French Minister of Health to investigate the field of clinical ethics in the United States and having spent 1 year in the MacLean Centre for Clinical Medical Ethics (Chicago) as a fellow in Mark Siegler's intensive training clinical ethics program. Her position led her to work on, among others, the ethical issues raised by concrete access to reproductive technologies on the clinical ground and to confront the way they were faced in France as opposed to the United States. In 2009, she published *Le bazar bioéthique* (The Bioethics Bazaar; Editions Robert Laffont, Paris) to alert readers to the difficulties encountered by couples who are not perfectly compliant with the norms of public morality in accessing such technologies, difficulties partly due to the illiberalism of the legislative framework to which the bioethics field is subject in France.

Lori Freedman, PhD, is Associate Professor of Obstetrics, Gynecology, and Reproductive Sciences at the University of California, San Francisco. She conducts qualitative research within the Advancing New Standards in Reproductive Health (ANSIRH) program. Dr. Freedman completed her sociology doctorate at the University of California, Davis, in 2008. She became a Greenwall Faculty Scholar in Bioethics in 2014 and an Emerging Leader in Health and Medicine at the National Academy of Medicine in 2017. Dr. Freedman investigates how reproductive healthcare is shaped by our medical institutions and social structures.

Melissa Gilliam, MD, MPH, is the Ellen H. Block Distinguished Service Professor of Health Justice and Vice Provost at the University of Chicago. Dr. Gilliam is the founder and director of the Center for Interdisciplinary Inquiry and Innovation in Sexual and Reproductive Health (Ci3), an interdisciplinary research center at the University of Chicago addressing the health of adolescents using technology, design, and narrative. She is also a member of the National Academy of Medicine. Her clinical focus is in pediatric and adolescent gynecology.

Valerie Gutmann Koch, JD, is Assistant Professor and Co-Director of the Health Law and Policy Institute at the University of Houston Law Center and Director of Law and Ethics at the MacLean Center for Clinical Medical Ethics at the University of Chicago. After receiving her law degree at Harvard Law School, Professor Koch was the Special Advisor and Senior Attorney to the New York State Task Force on Life and the Law, the state's bioethics commission. She has served as the Chair of the ABA's Special Committee on Bioethics and the Law and as Co-Chair of the Law Affinity Group for the American Society for Bioethics and the Humanities.

Lisa H. Harris, MD, PhD, is the F. Wallace and Janet Jeffries Collegiate Professor of Reproductive Health, Professor of Obstetrics and Gynecology, and Professor of Women's Studies at University of Michigan. After completing college and medical school at Harvard University, Dr. Harris completed obstetrics and gynecology residency at the University of California, San Francisco, and a PhD in American culture and women's studies at the University of Michigan. Her clinical work encompasses abortion, miscarriage, and birth care. She is known for interdisciplinary approaches to scholarship, including work on abortion stigma, experiences of abortion caregivers, conscience in reproductive healthcare, women's preferences for miscarriage management, and the social construction of assisted reproductive technologies. She serves as Associate Chair of her department and directs the University of Michigan's Fellowship in Complex Family Planning.

Lee Hasselbacher, JD, is Senior Policy Researcher at the Center for Interdisciplinary Inquiry and Innovation in Sexual and Reproductive Health (Ci3) at the University of Chicago. Lee leads Ci3's reproductive health policy research, collecting data and translating research to inform policy debates and legislation. Her research covers topics such as access to contraception and abortion, health insurance, religious refusals in healthcare, and consent and confidentiality for young people. Lee is a graduate of Northwestern Pritzker School of Law, where she focused on law and social policy, and the University of Wisconsin-Madison.

Timothy R. B. Johnson, MD, AM, FACOG, is Arthur F. Thurnau Professor of Obstetrics and Gynecology and Gender and Women's Studies and a member of the Center for Bioethics and Social Sciences in Medicine at the University of Michigan. His academic and clinical interests include fetal assessment, prenatal care, medical education and human resource capacity building, global women's health, reproductive justice, global health ethics, and assessment and prevention of sexual harassment in academic medicine. He has long been involved in international medical education and research, notably in Ghana, and is honorary Fellow of the West African College of Surgeons, the Ghana College of Physicians and Surgeons, and the Royal College of Obstetricians and Gynaecologists (London). He has received the Distinguished Service Award of the American College of Obstetricians and Gynecologists (ACOG), the Distinguished Merit Award of FIGO (International Federation of Gynecology and Obstetrics), and is an elected member of the US National Academy of Medicine.

Jhenifer Kliemchen Rodrigues, BSc, MSc, PhD, is Technical and Administrative Director at In Vitro Embriologia Clínica e Consultoria and Professor/Researcher at the Federal University, Minas Gerais, Brazil. Dr. Rodriques received her MS and PhD in biology of reproduction at the University of São Paulo and subsequently completed a postdoctoral fellowship in oncofertility at Oregon Health and Science University and a postdoctoral degree in molecular medicine at Federal University of Minas Gerais. She was a doctoral thesis winner of the CAPES Thesis Award, 2015 Edition, in the area of Medicine III and has published several scientific articles in this area. Dr. Rodriques is also a founding member of the Latin America Oncofertility Network and is a member of several medical societies, including the Brazilian Society for Reproductive Assistance (SBRA), the Brazilian Society for Human Reproduction (SBRH), Pronucleo, American Society for Reproductive Medicine (ASRM), and the European Society of Human Reproduction and Embryology (ESRHE). She has more than 16 years of experience in clinical embryology, research, and technical consultancy in reproductive medicine, having received merit certification in laboratory directorship, clinical embryology, and andrology by the Latin American Network for Assisted Reproduction (REDLARA).

Susan C. Klock, PhD, is a clinical psychologist specializing in the psychological aspects of assisted reproduction. She is Professor of Obstetrics and Gynecology and Psychiatry at Northwestern University's Feinberg School of Medicine. She provides consultation and counseling to individuals undergoing assisted reproduction treatment. She is past Chair of the Mental Health Professional Group of the American Society for Reproductive Medicine. Her program of research focuses on the psychosocial aspects of third-party reproduction. She has authored more than 50 peer-reviewed and invited publications regarding the psychological aspects of assisted reproduction and is current Specialty Editor for Mental Health, Ethics, and Sexuality for *Fertility and Sterility*.

Laurence B. McCullough, PhD, is Professor of Obstetrics and Gynecology, Zucker School of Medicine at Hofstra/Northwell at Lenox Hill Hospital in New York City and Distinguished Emeritus Professor in the Center for Medical Ethics and Health Policy, Baylor College of Medicine, Houston, Texas. After completing his doctorate in philosophy at the University of Texas at Austin, he was a Post-Doctoral Fellow at the Hastings Center. He has collaborated for 38 years with Dr. Frank A. Chervenak on ethics in obstetrics and gynecology, resulting in 286 peer-reviewed papers and three books. The most recent of these, co-authored with Dr. John H. Coverdale (Professor of Psychiatry and Medical Ethics, Baylor College of Medicine), *Professional Ethics in Obstetrics and Gynecology*, was published by Cambridge University Press in 2020.

Lynn M. Paltrow, JD, is the Founder and Executive Director of National Advocates for Pregnant Women. She is a graduate of Cornell University and New York University School of Law. Ms. Paltrow combines legal advocacy with grassroots and national organizing and policy work to secure the human and civil rights, health, and welfare of all people, focusing particularly on pregnant and parenting women and those who are most likely to be targeted for arrest and state control: women of color, low-income white women, and drug-using women. She has worked on numerous cases challenging restrictions on the right to choose abortion as well as cases opposing the prosecution of pregnant women seeking to continue their pregnancies to term. She is a frequent guest lecturer and writer for popular press, law reviews, and peer-reviewed journals.

Dorothy Roberts, JD, is the fourteenth Penn Integrates Knowledge Professor and George A. Weiss University Professor at the University of Pennsylvania, with joint appointments in the departments of Africana Studies and Sociology and the Law School, where she is the inaugural Raymond Pace and Sadie Tanner Mossell Alexander Professor of Civil Rights. She is also Founding Director of the Penn Program on Race, Science, and Society. Roberts has written and lectured extensively on law, public policy, and social justice issues related to reproductive freedom, child welfare, and bioethics. She is author of *Killing the Black Body: Race, Reproduction, and the Meaning of Liberty* (Pantheon, 1997/2017), *Shattered Bonds: The Color of Child Welfare* (Civitas, 2001), and *Fatal Invention: How Science, Politics, and Big Business Re-create Race in the Twenty-First Century* (New Press, 2011), and more than 100 scholarly articles and book chapters, as well as being co-editor of six books. Recent recognitions of her work include a 2019 election as a College of Physicians of Philadelphia Fellow, a 2017 election to the National Academy of Medicine, a 2016 Society of Family Planning Lifetime Achievement Award, a 2015 American Psychiatric Association Solomon Carter Fuller Award, and a 2011 election as a Hastings Center Fellow.

Heather E. Ross, JD, co-founded the law firm of Ross & Zuckerman, LLP, in 2005 to focus solely on legal issues surrounding assisted reproductive technology. Ms. Ross is a past chair to the Legal Professional Group of the American Society of Reproductive Medicine. She is also a member of the Academy of Adoption and Assisted Reproduction Attorneys, a professional member of Resolve, Family Equality Council, the LGBT Bar, and a committee member of the American Bar Association's Assisted Reproductive Technology Committee. Ms. Ross has represented thousands of clients in gamete donation, embryo donation, and gestational surrogacy arrangements. She is a frequent lecturer and writer in the area of assisted reproductive technology (ART) law and has presented numerous CLE courses to attorneys, medical professionals, and law students practicing in this field. Heather is also a Village Trustee in her hometown of Northbrook, Illinois, where she lives with her spouse, and 3 teenage girls—all of whom are the successful outcome of ART.

Kayte Spector-Bagdady, JD, MBe, is Associate Director at the Center for Bioethics and Social Sciences in Medicine and Assistant Professor of

Obstetrics and Gynecology at the University of Michigan Medical School. Professor Spector received her JD and master's degree in bioethics from the University of Pennsylvania Law School and School of Medicine, respectively, after graduating from Middlebury College. She served as Associate Director for President Obama's Presidential Commission for the Study of Bioethical Issues. She is currently on the Board of Directors for the American Society for Bioethics and Humanities.

David A. Strauss, BA, BPhil (Oxon), JD, is the Gerald Ratner Distinguished Service Professor of Law and Faculty Director of the Supreme Court and Appellate Clinic at the University of Chicago Law School, where he teaches and writes about constitutional law and related subjects. He has been a visiting professor at Harvard and Georgetown. He is the author of *The Living Constitution* (Oxford University Press, 2010), and he is an editor of the *Supreme Court Review.* He is a member of the American Academy of Arts and Sciences. He has been Assistant Solicitor General of the United States and Special Counsel to the US Senate Committee on the Judiciary.

Debra Stulberg, MD, MAPP, is Associate Professor and Chair of Family Medicine at the University of Chicago. She joined the University of Chicago faculty in 2007, with a primary appointment in Family Medicine and secondary appointments in the Obstetrics and Gynecology Section of Family Planning and Contraceptive Research, and the MacLean Center for Clinical Medical Ethics. Dr. Stulberg graduated from Harvard Medical School and completed her Family Medicine residency at West Suburban Hospital in Oak Park, Illinois. She received an MA in public policy from the University of Chicago, where she also completed fellowship training in primary care research and clinical medical ethics. Her research focuses on reproductive health service delivery in the United States. This includes studies on incorporating reproductive health in primary care, addressing racial and socioeconomic disparities in pregnancy outcomes, and understanding how religious healthcare institutions affect care delivery. She directs the Reproductive Health Outcomes and Disparities (RHOADs) Research Group and co-directs the Research Consortium on Religious Healthcare Institutions with co-author Lori Freedman. Dr. Stulberg provides patient care at a federally qualified health center on Chicago's south side.

Amber Truehart, MD, MSc, is Assistant Professor of Obstetrics and Gynecology at the University of Chicago. She completed her fellowship in family planning at the University of Chicago in 2015. She then completed specialized training in pediatric and adolescent gynecology and, in 2018, she received a Focused Practice Designation in Pediatric and Adolescent Gynecology from the American Board of Obstetrics and Gynecology (ABOG). Her clinical work focuses on hormonal counseling and management in adolescents with complex medical conditions. Dr. Truehart also serves as a member of the American College of Obstetricians and Gynecologists' Committee on Clinical Practice Guidelines–Gynecology.

Katie Watson, JD, is Associate Professor of Medical Social Sciences, Medical Education, and Obstetrics & Gynecology, and a Core Faculty Member of the Medical Humanities and Bioethics Graduate Program at Northwestern University's Feinberg School of Medicine (NU-FSM). Professor Watson is a graduate of NYU School of Law who clerked in the federal judiciary and worked in public interest law before completing Fellowships in Clinical Medical Ethics at the MacLean Center at the University of Chicago, and in Medical Humanities at NU-FSM. Her academic work focuses on women's health and reproductive ethics, and she is the author of *Scarlet A: The Ethics, Law, and Politics of Ordinary Abortion* (Oxford University Press, 2018). Professor Watson is currently on the National Abortion Federation Board of Directors, the National Medical Council of Planned Parenthood Federation of America, the Editorial Board of the AMA Journal of Ethics, and is a former Board member of the American Society for Bioethics and Humanities.

Teresa K. Woodruff, PhD, is Provost and Executive Vice President for Academic Affairs at Michigan State University. Prior to Michigan State, she was Thomas J. Watkins Professor of Obstetrics and Gynecology at the Feinberg School of Medicine, Director of the Center for Reproductive Science, Dean of the Graduate School at Northwestern University, and Founder and Director of the Oncofertility Consortium. She is an elected member of the National Academy of Medicine, American Academy of Arts and Science, National Academy of Inventors, and a recipient of a Guggenheim Fellowship.

Introduction

Julie Chor MD, MPH and Katie Watson JD

Like all clinicians, reproductive healthcare providers face specialty-specific ethical questions. However, the first editor of this book, Dr. Julie Chor (JC), an obstetrician-gynecologist who also completed a Complex Family Planning Fellowship, has never found an ethics text that is tailored to the needs of practicing clinicians, students, and trainees in reproductive healthcare. This is an unfortunate gap in the literature because whether reproductive health providers come from obstetrics and gynecology, family medicine, pediatrics, or another field, they all must be able to identify and analyze complex ethical issues that lie at the crossroads of patient decision-making, scientific advancement, political controversy, government regulation, and profound moral considerations in the context of continually evolving medical, legal, and societal factors. To fill this gap, Dr. Chor invited co-editor Professor Katie Watson (KW), a bioethics professor and lawyer who focuses on reproductive ethics, to partner in creating the text that she has always longed to use but has never found while practicing and teaching in this complex milieu.

This book is a carefully curated compilation of essays inspired by a lecture series at the University of Chicago's MacLean Center for Medical Ethics, where both JC and KW are former fellows, and JC is currently a faculty member. The essays are written by leading experts in the fields of ethics, medicine, law, and the social sciences addressing key issues in reproductive ethics. The book is organized into three sections: Contraception and Abortion Ethics: Preventing Pregnancy and Birth, Assisted Reproduction Ethics: Initiating Pregnancy, and Obstetric Ethics: Managing Pregnancy and Delivery. Each section begins with an overview by the editors that includes questions meant to inspire discussion about that section's essays. To maximize this book's usefulness to both trainees (including medical and nursing students, medical residents, and fellows) and experienced clinicians (including clinical ethicists, physicians, advanced practice nurses, nurse midwives, physician assistants, and social workers), we've kept the essays concise and we've ensured they avoid the trap of "neon light ethics"—ethical analysis of shocking or extraordinarily complex cases that almost never arise in actual practice. Instead they follow the model of the MacLean Center itself, analyzing the clinical ethics questions that routinely arise in the day-to-day practice of reproductive healthcare while also raising the "big picture" bioethics implications of our practice patterns and choices.

The contemporary lens of reproductive justice informs our bioethics approach throughout the book.[1] Reproductive justice connects people's right to sexuality without procreation (Section I), their right to have a baby (Sections II and III), and their right to parent the children they have (a topic often outside the scope of medical practice but implicated by essays like Flavin and Paltrow's analysis of breaking confidentiality to report pregnant patients to law enforcement). The reproductive justice framework also encourages us to focus on the needs and rights of the most marginalized. This approach is deserved as a matter of justice and, as a practical matter, it will typically also protect the needs and rights of those with higher incomes or more social capital. Justice is one of the traditional four principles of medical ethics analysis, and an emphasis on reproductive justice can make traditional principlism more robust by expanding it beyond the individual clinician–patient dyad and the snapshot of the clinical moment to include a longitudinal picture of the patient's lived experience in their intersectional identity and those groups' historical experience.

There are many frameworks for medical ethics, and advanced practitioners often find themselves consciously or unconsciously moving between them or combining them as situations seem to require. One foundational framework that explicitly or implicitly appears in numerous essays in this book (and is referenced in the preceding paragraph) is a framework of moral norms commonly referred to as "principlism" or the "four principles" framework, which was first described by Beauchamp and Childress in 1977.[2] Therefore, the four principles of autonomy, beneficence, nonmaleficence, and justice warrant brief definition here for readers who may be unfamiliar with them. The principle of *autonomy* refers to respect and support for individuals' ability and right to make and act on free, informed medical decisions.[2] The principle of *nonmaleficence*, the obligation to not cause harm, is frequently paired with the principle of *beneficence*, the obligation to act to help others.[2] The concept of *justice* encompasses the attempt to distribute benefits and burdens in a manner that is fair and equitable.[2,3] Principlism does not rank any of these principles as more important than another. Instead, it encourages clinicians to attend to each value, recognizing when they are in tension and balancing as possible or choosing as needed. When clinicians face scenarios that feel uncomfortable or ethically questionable for reasons that they are unable to clearly articulate, they should consider whether that is because two or more of these principles are in tension. Framing issues, problems, or questions in reproductive ethics through these principles often gives clinicians a way to parse their "gut reactions" to challenging encounters and to identify the root of a potential ethical conflict.

Books are divided in a way life often is not. We encourage readers to remember that the lines this book draws between preventing pregnancy, initiating pregnancy, and managing pregnancy can be crossed by the same individual, and many patients will be in each area more than once, bouncing between them from adolescence to menopause. They may also be dynamic in any one pregnancy: for example, a person who was initially trying to prevent pregnancy may choose to continue an unintended pregnancy, moving them from the prevention issue of Section I to the management issues of Section III, and, when faced with a diagnosis of fetal anomalies, that person might move back to the questions of pregnancy termination in Section I. This illustrates the need for specialists to maintain flexible mindsets across these phases— in the case just described, a maternal-fetal medicine (MFM) specialist must also be able to counsel like (and in some places, practice like) a family planning specialist. When a reproductive endocrinology and infertility (REI) specialist counsels someone seeking assistance getting pregnant (addressed in Section II), consideration of multiple embryo transfer requires them to look forward to the pregnancy management phase and think like an MFM. Or imagine a patient delivering by caesarian who wants a tubal ligation and is upset to learn that the fact that she is insured through Medicaid means she cannot have one because she did not consent 30 days before delivery. If she has attended prenatal care, this bad outcome may be the result of an obstetrician focused on delivery failing to also think like a family planning specialist and ask about her reproductive plans after this pregnancy and/or failing to provide care that is sensitive to her social context. (Medicaid requires advance consent for this family planning choice, and, because Medicaid covers some patients' medical costs during pregnancy and delivery but not afterward, delivery might be her only opportunity to have a wanted tubal.)

This book is meant to be illustrative, not comprehensive. It is not possible to cover every ethically challenging situation that can arise in reproductive healthcare provision. Similarly, we centered this book on reproduction and did not expand into other areas of sexual health and gynecologic ethics. Instead, we sought to provide frameworks and models of thinking that readers can take from the specific contexts described in these essays and apply to other situations not specifically addressed in this collection. When confronted with situations that are not directly addressed in this text, we urge readers to turn to the excellent work of colleagues at professional organizations that provide free, publicly available ethics opinions and position statements covering a wider spectrum of topics than can be addressed in this text, including the American College of Obstetricians and Gynecologists (ACOG), the American Society of Reproductive Medicine (ASRM), the American Academy of Family Physicians (AAFP), the American Academy of Pediatrics (AAP), and the Association of Women's Health, Obstetric, and Neonatal Nurses (AWHONN).

Language matters. The issues and concepts discussed in these essays apply to anyone with the capacity to become pregnant, a group that includes people who do not identify as female. We recognize and respect concerns around the use of gendered language and encourage readers to consider how language colors the ways in which we conceptualize ethical issues in reproductive healthcare provision, including throughout this text. However, readers will see that the words "woman" and "women" are sometimes used in these essays. Similarly, readers will note that essay authors use a variety of terms for the professionals to whom they refer, such "physicians," "providers," and "clinicians." We made an editorial choice to preserve each author's voice rather than imposing a standardizing format in these areas, in part because many write about past social or legal discrimination that hinged on a binary understanding of the abilities and roles of "women." However, regardless of the specific terminology that authors have chosen to use in their writing, as editors, we worked to make every essay relevant to the care of all people and instructive to both seasoned experts and trainees working in reproductive healthcare across disciplines such as nursing, social work, ethics, and medicine.

The cover image of a uterus is also meant to be inclusive, since a person with a uterus is the clinical focal point of pregnancy prevention, initiation, and management for people of all races, sexual orientations, and gender identities. The Exquisite Uterus project[4] invited over 200 artists to individualize a medical image of a uterus printed on fabric to communicate "My uterus is my own," and for us, Maggy Rozycki Hiltner's choice to do so with found antique embroidery connected the old "women's work" of sewing with the suturing done in the now majority-female profession of obstetrics and gynecology.

The luminaries who have shared their experience, intellect, and insight in the chapters of this book have also taught us a great deal, and we offer our heartfelt thanks to each for their patience. Their collective commitment to inquiry, advocacy, and pedagogy around some of today's most challenging issues in reproductive medicine is truly inspiring. We also thank the readers of this book for all they contribute every day. Both individually and as a collection, we hope these essays help you deliver the excellent, ethical care every patient seeking your support of their reproductive health deserves.

—Julie Chor and Katie Watson, November 3, 2020, Chicago, Illinois

Referneces

1. Ross LJ, Solinger R. *Reproductive Justice: An Introduction.* Berkeley: University of California Press; 2017.
2. Beauchamp TL, Childress JF. *Principles of Biomedical Ethics.* 8th ed. New York: Oxford University Press; 2019.
3. Johnson AR, Siegler M, Winslade WJ. *Clinical Ethics: A Practical Approach to Ethical Decisions in Clinical Medicine.* 8th ed. New York: McGraw-Hill Education; 2015.
4. http://exquisiteuterus.com

SECTION I
CONTRACEPTION AND ABORTION ETHICS

Preventing Pregnancy and Birth

Overview

Contraception and Abortion Ethics

Katie Watson JD and Julie Chor MD, MPH

The ethics of family planning invokes both bioethics, which are ethical issues relevant to groups of patients and/or society at large, and clinical ethics, which are the daily decisions affecting the care of individual patients.

This section's first chapter invites clinicians to root their family planning practice in the big-picture perspective of bioethics, with physician Melissa Gilliam and law professor Dorothy Roberts arguing that we must understand the concept of reproductive justice before we can analyze reproductive ethics. "Reproductive freedom" has typically meant the right to not have a child. "Reproductive justice" is a more holistic concept that connects the right to not have a child, the right to have a child, and the right to parent and centers the needs and experiences of the most marginalized. Gilliam and Roberts focus on the principle of justice by reminding us that "women" are not a homogenous group and by reviewing efforts to regulate the reproduction of women of color differently or more extremely than the reproduction of white women. But their ultimate focus is on the clinical ethics of contemporary patient–provider interactions, and their goal is to help clinicians avoid coercive behaviors, better understand patient perspectives, and seek opportunities to examine their own assumptions as well as the structural inequalities that remain unaddressed by the choice framework.

Then we move from the impact of the patient's race on family planning to the impact of the provider's religion. In Chapter 2, physician Debra Stulberg and sociologist Lori Freedman go beyond the familiar question of clinician conscience to analyze the consequences of "institutional conscience." More than 1 in 5 hospital beds in the United States are located in a religiously affiliated hospital (in some states the number is nearly half), and 70% of these are Catholic. However, medical organizations like the American College of Obstetricians and Gynecologists (ACOG) and the American Medical Association (AMA) have not yet issued ethics guidelines defining the obligations of *institutions* that refuse to provide care, as opposed to the obligations of individual clinicians. When an institution prohibits its clinicians from providing legal, standard-of-care family planning services that the patient and clinician think are ethically and medically appropriate, how can patients be protected from discrimination? Stulberg and Freedman urge us to see this as an issue of informed decision making: for example, they argue that it is unethical for a patient seeking tubal ligation at the time of caesarian delivery to be surprised to learn she will have to incur the expense and risk of scheduling a second surgery elsewhere or for a patient to unknowingly receive miscarriage management that risks her health in order to preserve a religious hospital's "conscience." Instead, they provide a guide for clinicians working in private groups, clinics, or hospitals owned by these systems, and they advocate for greater public transparency about religiously limited healthcare organizations in order to spare patients who do not share these institutions' perspectives burdens like these.

In Chapter 3, physician Amber Truehart, policy researcher Lee Hasselbacher, and physician-ethicist Julie Chor do a deep dive into clinical ethics, focusing on minors and a too-often overlooked issue in their reproductive healthcare: confidentiality. They begin by illuminating the public health imperatives behind laws allowing minors to consent to their own reproductive healthcare (as opposed to the rights-based rationales that drove laws protecting adults' reproductive healthcare), then they point out a crucial gap: the legal right to consent to healthcare usually comes with a right to confidentiality, but the current structure of our medical systems and insurance protocols often breaks that link for minors. Clinicians who do not understand these factors risk making false promises to vulnerable patients, robbing them of information (whether their care will or will not be disclosed to their parents) that is material to their consent process. Therefore, these adolescent health experts educate clinicians about systems issues that can breach confidentiality, instruct clinicians how to advocate for their patients by anticipating and overcoming these barriers, and counsel for transparency with adolescent patients when issues like insurance billing practices or the structure of your clinic's electronic medical record mean you cannot actually guarantee confidentiality.

This is an ethics book, yet because legislatures and courts have played a huge role in defining whether family planning professionals and their patients can do what both believe is ethical, law professor David Strauss's overview of the regulation of abortion and contraception in the United States (Chapter 4) is essential. This accessible essay helps clinicians understand the constitutional reasoning that led to both the right to contraception and the right to abortion, and it gives them the legislative history they need to put today's headlines in context. The confirmation of Justice Amy Coney Barrett as the replacement for Justice Ruth Bader Ginsburg throws many Supreme Court precedents into question, and this foundational chapter will help readers make sense of any changes to come as well.

However, because the law of abortion has loomed so largely over the practice of abortion, here we offer some analysis of the ethics of abortion. In our experience, people who provide and receive abortion care often allow discussion of what is legal to displace discussion of what is ethical. Sometimes it is because they believe abortion is obviously and indisputably ethical, but they struggle to find language for explaining why. Other times, it's because they believe discussion of the moral status of embryos and fetuses is an insincere cover for an unspoken claim that women should not be allowed the power of sexual or reproductive control, and this makes them reluctant to engage in discussions about "the ethics of abortion" as opposed to "the rights of women." Regardless of the reasons for it, pro-choice people's silence on the topic can create a false impression that opponents of these medical technologies and procedures are the only ones thinking about ethics.

Therefore, we think it is important to articulate something that is obvious to many people in this field: that clinicians who provide and patients who choose to receive contraception or abortion typically do so because they are moral agents who have concluded that contraception and/or abortion are either morally acceptable or morally good. Morality is often equated with religion in abortion care, yet mainstream medical ethics has become a largely secular enterprise in the United States. Therefore, it can be useful to articulate how the traditional medical ethics analysis of principlism supports access to abortion.[1]

The principlist analysis of abortion must address nonmaleficence: Does abortion "do harm" to a person or a patient? People who think abortion is morally acceptable say it does not because they reject what abortion opponents call the "substantial identity" argument: that people are intrinsically valuable because of what we are, and what we are is a physical organism that comes to be at conception because a fertilized egg contains the genetic blueprint for a human being.[2] (A religious version of this argument substitutes "soul" for "DNA.") Instead, people who conclude abortion is morally acceptable think that qualities gained during pregnancy, such as the ability to think, feel, or survive outside the womb, are required to turn human tissue into a human being. They rarely claim that an embryo's potential to become a person (or its "latent qualities") is of no importance. But they also reject the potentiality argument, which says embryos and fetuses must be given the same value of what they have the potential to become, which is people.[3] Just as potentiality does not give an acorn the same value as an oak tree, those who think abortion is morally acceptable conclude that it is morally right to put embryos and people in different categories.

Substantial identity and potentiality arguments often include a claim that a fertilized egg contains everything it needs to become a person. This is incorrect. To become a person, it also must be nourished by, and make a bloody exit from, a woman. This fact leads some to conclude that the central moral feature of pregnancy is that human development must take place inside a person's body. Assigning rational, sentient, biologically independent women a higher moral status than biologically dependent embryos or fetuses leads to the conclusion that forced childbearing is immoral and that a woman's decision to end an unwanted pregnancy is a morally acceptable act.

Concluding that abortion does not violate the principle of nonmaleficence makes it morally acceptable. This view explains why many pro-choice people see conception as a moral invitation rather than a moral obligation. "Moral" because whether to bring a child into the world is a value-laden decision of tremendous consequence to human health and happiness, and "invitation" because pregnancy is an opportunity for motherhood that one may accept or decline.

Another secular ethics position is that abortion is morally good. This view is held by the healthcare professionals who provide abortion care—they would not make it part or all of their life's work if they believed otherwise— and it is supported by the traditional medical ethics principles of autonomy, beneficence, and justice.

Clinicians who provide abortions honor the medical ethics principle of autonomy by helping their patients preserve bodily integrity, decisional freedom, and the dignity of dominion over their life's course. Childbearing dramatically alters a woman's identity and life experience, and, in the United States, childbirth carries a risk of death about 14 times higher than abortion.[4] When a woman does not see enduring pregnancy and delivering a child as a benefit, an autonomy analysis respects her as a moral agent who is following her values and allows her to decline the physical and social risks of childbearing.

Clinicians who provide abortions honor the medical ethics principle of beneficence by preventing the harms of forced childbearing and unsafe abortion. The principle of beneficence also illuminates some patients' abortion decisions as an expression of a mother's love. In the United States, 59% of abortion patients already have one or more children,[5] and commitment to meeting their existing children's needs can contribute to their decision to decline nature's invitation to nurture another embryo to fruition. Similarly, when a young woman believes she can't yet be the kind of mother she wants her children to have, her abortion might be a beneficent act toward her future children.

Clinicians who provide abortions honor the medical ethics principle of justice in two ways. Abortion access is a component of economic justice because parenthood is expensive. In the United States, 49% of abortion patients have incomes below the poverty line and an additional 26% have low incomes[6]; 73% of abortion patients list "can't afford a baby now" as one of their reasons, and 23% list it as "the most important reason."[7] Until society ensures the economic and social conditions needed to support childrearing, allowing low-income women and families the option of abortion prevents them from being pushed even further into poverty.

Abortion access is also essential to gender justice. Women have long been subjected to legal and social discrimination on the basis of their biological capacity for pregnancy. Today, the relatively new medical technologies of safe, effective contraception and abortion allow women to escape pregnancy's physical and social impact and to come close to men's degree of sexual and reproductive freedom. Women cannot have social, economic, and interpersonal power comparable to men unless they can control whether and when they have children. Therefore, women's moral claim to equal opportunity requires access to abortion for pregnant women who want it.

Some people's opposition to contraception is grounded in the same perspective that leads them to oppose abortion: a belief that it is unethical to do anything that might destroy a fertilized egg, including preventing implantation. Individuals who adhere to this perspective, therefore, consider intrauterine devices (IUDs) to be "abortifacients." Other opposition to contraception is grounded in beliefs about the ethics of sexuality. For example, the Catholic Church takes the position that it is immoral for people to engage in any sex outside of marriage, and any sex within marriage when the parties are not at least open to procreation. Therefore, the Church opposes contraception because it "contradicts the full truth of the sexual act as the proper expression of conjugal love" and because contraception "is opposed to the virtue of chastity in marriage."[8] This position is enforced by the Ethical and Religious Directives (ERDs) governing Catholic healthcare, which prohibit their clinicians from providing contraceptives or sterilizing procedures.[9]

A principlist analysis in support of access to contraception parallels many of the arguments in support of access to abortion. In contrast to those who have moral or ethical objections to contraception, those who believe contraception is morally neutral or morally good typically believe that sex between consenting parties is morally neutral or morally good. Alternatively, they may believe that intercourse is morally bad (in general, or in a particular instance) but that withholding contraceptives is unlikely to stop that intercourse from happening and that allowing an unwanted pregnancy to result from that act would only make a bad situation worse. Accordingly, clinicians who provide contraception not only reject the notion that this care is harmful, thereby adhering to the principle of nonmaleficence, but also view this care as promoting their patients' well-being, thereby fulfilling their commitment to beneficence. Because contraception allows individuals to prevent pregnancy and, therefore, exert control over their life course, providing contraception also supports individuals' autonomy. Similarly, by providing individuals with tools to determine if, when, and under what circumstances to become pregnant, ensuring and expanding access to contraception fosters economic and gender justice.

Retaining respect and compassion for patients who see the world differently than you do is central to the practice of medicine. All clinicians should learn what scope of services their patient finds morally acceptable and ensure their patient has the information relevant to their moral framework. For example, a patient who believes it is unacceptable for her to disrupt a fertilized egg will need details about the mechanisms of different contraceptive options in order to engage in informed decision-making, and a patient who does not hold this belief might prefer to focus on efficacy and ease of use. In our pluralistic society, the same is true of the need for reciprocal respect between colleagues. Political attacks on the character of clinicians who provide abortions in the United States have created an urgent need to communicate that every physician is a moral agent engaged in ethical decision-making and acts of conscience in partnership with patients.

Discussion Questions

Chapter 3: Gilliam and Roberts, "Why Reproductive Justice Matters to Reproductive Ethics"
What role can you play in dismantling oppression? How might an intentional shift toward working within a reproductive justice framework change your clinical choices? Does understanding the concept of reproductive justice change your analysis of reproductive ethics?

Chapter 4: Freedman and Stulberg, "Religiously Affiliated Healthcare Institutions: An Ethical Analysis of What They Mean for Patients, Clinicians, and Our Health System"
Do you work in a religiously affiliated institution? If yes, do you know all the limitations on your practice? Do your patients know these limitations? If not, do you agree that you should tell your patients these limitations up front, even if it might lead to a loss of income? The ACOG Ethics Opinion on Conscience says "In the provision of reproductive services, the patient's well-being must be paramount. Any conscientious refusal that conflicts with a patient's well-being should be accommodated only if the primary duty to the patient can be fulfilled."[10] What could or should religious affiliated health-care organizations do to support patient autonomy? If they refuse to take these steps, why do you think that is?

Chapter 5: Truehart, Hasselbacher, and Chor, "Contemporary Challenges to Providing Confidential Reproductive Healthcare to Minors"
Can you promise your minor patients true confidentiality? What are the barriers to this in your practice setting? What could you do to reduce or elim-inate these barriers? If barriers remain, how will you integrate this fact into your minor counseling and consent process?

Chapter 6: Strauss, "Contraception and Abortion in the United States: A Brief Legal History"
Where does the "right to privacy" come from? What was the rationale for finding a constitutional right to use contraception? How was that related to finding a constitutional right to abortion? How did *Casey* limit *Roe*, and in what way did *Whole Women's Health* modify or elaborate on *Casey*? What role has the AMA played in American abortion legislation?

References

1. Adapted from Watson K. Abortion as a moral good. *Lancet*. 2019;393(March 23):1196–97.
2. E.g., Lee P. The pro-life argument from substantial identity: A defence. *Bioethics*. 2004;18(3):249–63; Beckwith FJ. The explanatory power of the substance view of persons. *Christian Bioethics*. 2004;10(1):33–54.
3. E.g., Engelhardt Jr HT. The ontology of abortion. *Ethics*. 1974;84(3):217–34; Wade FC. Potentiality in the abortion discussion. *Rev Metaphysics*. 1975;239–55; Parness JA, Pritchard SK. To be or not to be: Protecting the unborn's potentiality of life. *U Cincinnati Law Rev*. 1982;51:257.
4. Raymond EG, Grimes DA. The comparative safety of legal induced abortion and childbirth in the United States. *Obstet Gynecol*. 2012;119:215–19.
5. Guttmacher Institute, Fact Sheet: Induced Abortion in the United States. 2019 Sep, https://www.guttmacher.org/fact-sheet/induced-abortion-united-states
6. Jerman J, Jones RK, Onda T. *Characteristics of U.S. Abortion Patients in 2014 and Changes Since 2008*. New York: Guttmacher Institute; 2016, https://www.guttmacher.org/report/characteristics-us-abortion-patients-2014.
7. Finer LB, Frohwirth LF, Dauphinee LA, Singh S, Moore AM. Reasons U.S. women have abortions: Quantitative and qualitative perspectives. *Perspect Sex Reprod Health*. 2005;37(3):110–18.
8. Pope John Paul II, 1995 Encyclical. Ioannes Paulus PP. II, *Evangelium Vitae* (March 25, 1995), http://w2.vatican.va/content/john-paul-ii/en/encyclicals/documents/hf_jp-ii_enc_25031995_evangelium-vitae.html.
9. "Catholic health institutions may not promote or condone contraceptive practices but should provide, for married couples and the medical staff who counsel them, instruction both about the Church's teaching on responsible parenthood and in methods of natural family planning." *United States Conference of Catholic Bishops, Ethical and Religious Directives for Catholic Health Care Services*, 6th ed. (2018), Directive 52.
10. Committee on Ethics. "The limits of conscientious refusal in reproductive medicine." ACOG Committee Opinion 385, November 2007.

1

Why Reproductive Justice Matters to Reproductive Ethics

Melissa Gilliam MD, MPH and Dorothy Roberts JD

Introduction

This chapter focuses on reproductive justice in the United States as it pertains to Black, brown, and Indigenous women (i.e., women of color) who have a long history of resistance to the devaluation and policing of their reproductive lives. It is essential that clinicians know this history as it continues to affect reproductive healthcare and underlie ongoing mistrust between women of color and the healthcare system. We see this history in enslaved African women's acts of rebellion against slaveholders' control of their childbearing. It continues through struggles in the 1960s for state recognition of welfare rights to ensure public assistance for families and through Black and brown women's campaigns in the 1970s for government regulations to prevent rampant sterilization abuse. The work of Black feminist theorizing, such as the Combahee River Collective's 1977 statement about the ways that interlocking systems of oppression affect people's status and experiences has contributed intellectual grounding for conceiving of these historical instances as a longer history of struggle.

Today, this struggle is referred to under the heading of *reproductive justice*. The term "reproductive justice" was coined in 1994 by 12 US-based Black women in two major precipitating events: a June 1994 conference in Chicago sponsored by the Illinois Pro-Choice Alliance and the Ms. Foundation for Women, and the September 1994 International Conference on Population and Development in Cairo, Egypt.[1] Since then, the intellectual tradition of reproductive justice has expanded to account for the needs of women in the Global South and has absorbed intellectual influences ranging from the human rights framework to the African philosophical tradition of Ubuntu.[2] The scope and mission of reproductive justice has been forwarded by organizations such as the SisterSong Women of Color Reproductive Justice Collective and, in recent years, been defined and clarified in writings by the movement's central figures.[3–5]

At its core, the reproductive justice framework can be formulated as three interconnected rights: the right to *have* a child (under the conditions chosen by the one having the child), the right *not* to have a child (if those conditions are not met), and the right to *parent* any children that one has. The second of those rights—the right not to have a child—aligns the reproductive justice framework broadly with the "pro-choice" movement of (white) American feminism. However, the reproductive justice framework differs from the more commonly used concept of reproductive choice in important, and radical, ways.

At this current historical juncture, the language of "choice" dominates the discussion of family planning, reproductive rights, and reproductive ethics. Advocates of abortion access have, for decades, described their position as "pro-choice," framing the opposing position as unnecessary government intrusion into the choices women should be able to make on their own. The adoption of the "choice" framing of access to reproductive care was an act of political triangulation and by no means a value-neutral decision. In choosing this framing, abortion rights advocates of the 1970s and 1980s made a calculated move to adopt a "fundamentally conservative approach," one built on the notion of restricting government interference in women's lives rather than creating the social conditions necessary for women's freedom.[3] As Jael Silliman points out, the "choice" language reflects a "neoliberal tradition that locates individual rights at its core."[6] The mainstream reproductive rights movement adopted a "choice" framework because it was seen as politically expedient at the time, and this framework has enjoyed subsequent longevity. However, it is insufficient to address the history and current realities of women of color and has been harmful to the cause of advancing reproductive freedom for all women. The reproductive justice framework serves as a useful corrective, challenging and transcending the "pro-choice" rhetoric that (white) feminist discourse in the United States has ossified into.

The rhetoric of "choice" predominantly privileges white upper and middle-class women who have the ability to choose from reproductive options that are unavailable to poor and low-income women, especially women of color. To echo Silliman, the "pro-choice" language "obscures the social context in which individuals make choices, and discounts the ways in which the state regulates populations, disciplines individual bodies, and exercises control over sexuality, gender, and reproduction."[6] The choice framing therefore proves useless for claiming public resources that most women need for their well-being and in order to freely make decisions about their bodies and their lives. Indeed, giving women "choices" has weakened the argument for state support because women without sufficient resources are simply held responsible for making "bad" choices.

Fundamentally, the choice framework fails to acknowledge the historical and current attempts to regulate and devalue the reproduction of Black women through ideologies, policies, and practices that encourage the oppressive use of contraception. At its most extreme, this history has included sterilization and forced contraception, conducted as part of the eugenics movement within the United States. Although few would defend or claim the lineage of eugenics today, echoes of its logic remain in such efforts as the promotion of long-acting reversible contraception (LARC) for "risky" populations. Ironically, efforts to regulate Black women's reproduction through pressure to use certain types of contraception coincide with a lack of access to abortion and safe motherhood. It is for this reason that the reproductive justice framework incorporates its two other rights: the right to *have* a child and the right to *parent* any children that one has. Expanding beyond the ideological framing of "pro-choice" language, these additional rights directly confront the history of white supremacy and the historical role that state-sponsored eugenics, forced sterilization, and punitive measures against mothers have played in denying women of color their rights to informed reproductive self-determination.

These topics are often omitted from discussions about reproductive ethics—and, simultaneously, social justice is often neglected as a major ethical principle. Yet, in order for women of color to have a different experience of reproductive healthcare, a discussion of reproductive justice must be centered. This chapter will discuss major topics in family planning and maternal health from the perspective of reproductive justice. "Reproductive justice" provides an alternative to the "choice" framing, one that can better account for the historical impact that white supremacy has had on the ability of women of color to make informed and consensual decisions about their reproductive health. Approaching Black women's reproductive freedom from a reproductive justice perspective offers an important way to expand our understanding of reproductive ethics. In doing so, it is our intent to add to the existing literature on reproductive ethics an analysis of reproductive freedom for Black women as it relates to family planning (contraception and abortion) and maternal mortality from a reproductive justice perspective. This chapter also provides essential information for clinicians who wish to improve the reproductive health of women of color by placing current clinical debates in a historical context.

The Medical Profession's Role in Perpetuating Reproductive Injustice

The genesis of the reproductive justice movement is closely linked to the history of reproductive medicine in the United States. Not only is the medical profession not immune to bias, but medical professionals also have been among the main perpetrators of oppressive practices.

The Origins of Gynecology

James Marion Sims, born January 1813, is known as the "father of modern gynecology." Among his many accolades, he is credited for developing the surgical technique to repair fistulous tracts, or passages, between the vagina and rectum or vagina and bladder that occur due to traumatic births or surgery. Yet it is less commonly taught that he developed his techniques using enslaved Black women. He reported operations on 12 enslaved women with fistulas, including one named Anarcha on whom he operated 13 times before he was successful. His activities included experimentation, complications, and reoperations, and he did not use anesthesia during the procedure.[7] These practices represent the understanding of that time: Black women were considered less than human and lacking any rights to bodily autonomy.

Eugenics in the United States

The reproductive justice movement partially arose as a reaction to the history of eugenics in the United States and the use of sterilization to control the reproduction of poor women and women of color. In some states, state-sponsored sterilization was used to prevent procreation by people with mental illness, alcoholism, or others it deemed "feeble-minded." Physicians performed more than 60,000 forced sterilizations in government-sponsored programs.[8,9] In states such as North Carolina, public welfare departments could petition for sterilization of their clients. While there are reports of some women requesting state-funded sterilization because they no longer desired fertility, the state also authorized involuntary sterilization for the "public good," resulting in the sterilization of perhaps more than 7,000 individuals by the Eugenics Board of North Carolina. In 2013, the North Carolina legislature passed a bill approving reparations. In 1976, the US Department of Health, Education, and Welfare developed measures to prevent sterilization coercion. These measures included prohibiting the sterilizing of young women and of women with mental disabilities, adding waiting periods between consent and sterilization, and drafting a standard consent form.[10] The contemporary push to remove mandated waiting periods for sterilization among recipients of Medicaid may lack a historical awareness of why these types of safeguards were put in place. Similarly, while some have argued that these laws prevent women from getting desired care, coercive practices still continue. From 2006 to 2010, more than 140 incarcerated women were sterilized in California prisons. Prison, as an institution, impairs autonomy, and many of these women described being pressured to undergo sterilization.[11,12]

Oppressive Policies and Practices of LARC Prescription in the Shadow of Eugenics

The coercive prescription of contraception for poor women and women of color also extends to modern methods of reversible contraception, including injectable and implantable contraception. While reproductive justice supports women having access to contraception, medical providers and policymakers have also played a role in overusing reversible contraception. Norplant was a six-rod implantable, progestin-only method of contraception providing 5 years of contraceptive efficacy accompanied by the absence of menses. Norplant was first marketed in 1991 in the United States in the face of rising teenage pregnancy rates, and was considered a major breakthrough, being one of the first new major methods of contraception in 30 years. Family planning advocates began to see Norplant as a possible solution to the rise in the rate of unintended and teenage pregnancy that had occurred in the 1980s.[13] A (now infamous) editorial in the *Philadelphia Inquirer* drew a link between the arrival of Norplant and poverty among Black children, suggesting that Norplant could be used to break the cycle of urban poverty in the United States.[14] Before long, courts were ordering Norplant use, and 13 states were openly considering incentivizing women for its use. Finally, the Indian Health Service was found to have distributed depo-medroxy progesterone acetate—an injectable contraceptive lasting 3 months—and later Norplant with minimal counseling or explanation of its benefits and risks.[15]

The Prosecution of Black Mothers

In the late 1980s, prosecutors around the country began to charge women with crimes for using drugs while pregnant. Between 1985 and 1995, at least 200 women in 30 states were charged with maternal drug use, the vast majority of whom were poor and Black and addicted to crack cocaine.[13] The medical profession played a significant role in turning the health problem of substance use during pregnancy into a crime. Doctors and nurses both helped to portray substance use by pregnant patients as despicable conduct that warranted criminal punishment and facilitated their patients' arrest and incarceration. The identification of a "crack epidemic" in the 1980s coincided with a 1988 study by the National Association for Perinatal Addiction Research and Education that found that 11% of newborns in 36 hospitals surveyed were affected by their mothers' illegal drug use during pregnancy. Policymakers and the media located both problems in Black communities and created a panic over gestational crack cocaine exposure.

Building on a long-standing, disparaging mythology about Black mothers as dangerous reproducers, the media depicted mothers addicted to crack cocaine as careless and selfish women who put their love for drugs above concern for their children.[13]

The media also created the so-called crack baby—typically assumed to be Black, although use of crack and other illegal drugs cut across racial categories—who was described not only as suffering permanent physical damage but as lacking any social consciousness. Medical professionals contributed to this false portrait of pregnant crack addicts and their babies. Medical journals focused one-sided attention on studies showing detrimental outcomes from cocaine exposure, and doctors and nurses repeated stereotypes about the effects to newspaper reporters. In fact, subsequent medical research has discredited the disparaging portrayal of the "crack baby" as scientifically unfounded.

In addition to being complicit in making gestational drug exposure a crime, applied largely along racial lines, the medical profession helped to target Black women for prosecution. Testing for and reporting of positive infant toxicologies were performed almost exclusively in public hospitals that served poor minority communities.[13] Private hospitals were less likely to have drug screening protocols and rarely reported their patients to the police. Several studies showed that medical staff were far more likely to report Black women who used drugs during pregnancy than their white patients. A 1990 study in Pinellas County, Florida, for example, discovered that doctors were 10 times more likely to report Black women than white women to government authorities despite similar rates of substance use. This illustrates how the medical profession continues to be complicit in creating and enforcing policies that punish Black mothers for having children rather than making the social changes needed for their patients' freedom and well-being.

Welfare Restructuring and Family Caps

The Personal Responsibility and Work Opportunity Reconciliation Act (PRWORA), passed by Congress and signed into law by President Clinton in 1996, abolished the federal entitlement to welfare. In place of guaranteeing public assistance to struggling families, the law instituted a behavior modification program aimed at regulating the reproductive decisions of cash-poor mothers.[16] Key to these policies are workfare rules that force recipients into low-wage jobs as well as provisions punishing their childbearing and pressuring them to get married. The policy shift was fueled by stereotypes of Black women, especially the "Welfare Queen"—promoted initially by the Reagan Administration—who was portrayed as breeding children just to fatten her welfare check and then wasting the money recklessly on herself.

In the wake of welfare restructuring, many states have passed "child exclusions" or "family caps" that aim to deter women receiving public assistance from having babies by denying them any increment in their benefits, thus infringing their reproductive autonomy and denying their families income needed to survive.[16] Congress noted in its 2001 Temporary Assistance for Needy Families (TANF) reauthorization bill that "[s]tates in which African Americans make up a higher proportion of recipients are statistically more likely to adopt family cap policies," and studies have found that caps influenced Black women's reproductive decisions the most out of all women.

Long-Term Disparities: Maternal and Infant Morbidity and Mortality

The historical injustices just discussed have left their mark in the form of lingering health disparities. Black women are three to four times more likely than white women to die due to pregnancy-related complications. Out of those Black women who do die from complications to pregnancy, 44% of them have medically preventable deaths, as opposed to only 30% of white women.[17] In 2014, Black mothers experienced an infant mortality rate of 1,104 deaths per 100,000 live births, compared to 492 deaths per 100,000 live births for white mothers.[18] In 2015, 13.41% of births to Black mothers and 9.14% of births to Hispanic mothers were preterm, as opposed to 8.88% of births to white mothers.[19]

Contraceptive use among Black women lags behind contraceptive use among white women: 83% of Black women at risk of unintended pregnancy uses contraception versus 91% of white women.[20] This lower incidence of contraceptive use correlates with a higher incidence of abortion: in 2014, the abortion rate among Black women was roughly 2.7 times higher than that of white women, and the abortion rate among Hispanic women was roughly 1.7 times higher.[21] As one might expect, this higher abortion rate reflects a higher rate of unintended pregnancy: data from 2008 indicated that 70% of pregnancies among Black women and 57% of pregnancies among Hispanic women were unintended, standing in contrast to 42% of pregnancies among white women.[22]

The rates of sexually transmitted infections also remain higher for women of color than for their white counterparts. In 2016, the rate of reported cases of chlamydia, gonorrhea, and primary and secondary syphilis for Black women were 5.1 times, 8.4 times, and 7.0 times the rate of reported cases for white women, respectively. Reported gonorrhea cases among American Indian and Alaskan Native women were 6.1 times the rates of white women, and those of Native Hawaiian and Pacific Islanders were 3.4 times that of white women. Reported gonorrhea cases among Hispanic women were 1.6 times the rates of white women.[23]

Finally, some women of color experience higher rates of sexual assault than their white counterparts. Sexual assault victimization rates between 2005 and 2010, as reported by the US Department of Justice Bureau of Justice Statistics, were slightly higher for Black women (2.8 per 1,000) than for white women (2.2 per 1,000). Native American and Alaskan Native women suffered from especially disproportionate rates of sexual assault, at 4.4 per 1,000.[24]

Implications for Policy and Practice

Achieving the three interconnected rights encompassed by reproductive justice requires supporting individual freedoms as well as addressing social, political, and systemic inequities that limit individual reproductive freedom. This multisystem or socioecological perspective accounts for the context and conditions in which individuals live. Ecological models describe the individual within a larger social and political milieu: disparities in health outcomes are not merely a reflection of health behaviors or choice, but instead reflect social, political, and structural factors that limit personal freedom. Such factors include but are not limited to access to quality healthcare, good schools, safe streets, well-paying jobs, clean water, and quality foods. It is clear how the absence of each of these factors limits one's ability to form a family of one's choosing. Ecological frameworks help to indicate the many factors that can be addressed to further reproductive justice. Such an integrated model is critical for linking reproductive healthcare practice to policy.

Thus, reproductive justice is more than a critique of the status quo. It is a powerful approach to working toward improving the reproductive lives of individuals marginalized by their color, ethnicity, disability status, or sexual or gender identity. As such, it can be useful for healthcare providers and policymakers to integrate in their thinking, practice, and advocacy.

The rising rates of maternal mortality and preterm birth that disproportionately affect poor women and communities of color suggest that our current model of focusing intensely on prenatal care is an inadequate model of healthcare. Lu and Halfon argue for the need to examine differential exposures to risk and protective factors not just during pregnancy, but over the life course of women. Thus, interventions and policies that are longitudinal and take into account context are needed to change these outcomes.[25]

Reproductive justice also has implications for contraceptive practices and policies. The history of forced sterilization in the United States resulted in a mandated 30-day waiting period between the time a woman who is insured by Medicaid signs a consent form for sterilization and the time she receives sterilization. Numerous studies have demonstrated that many women who request sterilization do not undergo the procedure for a myriad of reasons, including changing their minds or lack of valid sterilization consent forms at the time of delivery. The latter problem has caused many to argue for abolishing the forms as biased against poor women. This particular solution is blunt and may prevent some women from obtaining a desired procedure due to hospital logistics and other unintended barriers. Yet the continuing legacy of devaluing childbearing by women of color, especially if they are poor, shows that there is a need for additional clinical safeguards to prevent the coercive use of sterilization among poor women.

The past two decades have seen the emergence of the intrauterine device and the contraceptive implant, two forms of highly effective contraception that, unlike sterilization, are reversible. LARCs are the most effective methods of contraception because they require fewer use behaviors. These methods are an important source of reproductive freedom for women who choose them, so it is crucial that women have access to these methods without being fettered by the 2-day clinic visit or issues of availability.[26,27] Nevertheless, as in the case of sterilization, there is a need for high-quality care free from the coercion or bias practiced by some clinicians and policymakers in the case of Norplant. To that end, the National Women's Health Network-SisterSong joint Statement of Principles on LARC was created to guide clinicians and others in providing LARC care for women. These groups urge that LARC should be offered as one of many options but that women should not be guided to these methods in particular.

More broadly, healthcare professionals and policymakers should oppose policies that blame and punish marginalized women's childbearing for the disadvantages experienced by their children that are actually caused by structural inequalities. In recent years, the prosecution of women for fetal crimes has been facilitated by state fetal protection laws that directly criminalize pregnant women by giving fetuses the same legal status as an already born child.[16] For example, Alabama revised its homicide laws in 2006 to include "an unborn child in utero at any stage of development, regardless of viability" as a "person" or "human being." In 2014, Tennessee became the first state in the nation to pass a law making it a crime for women to use illegal narcotics while pregnant. The criminalization of pregnant women is taking place in the context of a growing carceral state that incarcerates increasing numbers of mothers—who themselves are survivors of violence, addiction, and abuse—for nonviolent offenses.

At the same time, state programs that provide resources and other supports to struggling mothers have been decimated. A reproductive justice approach calls clinicians to work against policies that respond to women's marginalization by punishing them; instead, we should work toward replacing punitive approaches with policies such as universal healthcare—including high-quality abortion, contraceptive, prenatal, and birthing care—and alternatives to prison that generously support the reproductive freedom and well-being of everyone.

Conclusion

Reproductive justice is a powerful lens that helps to reframe those considerations of health that have stalled because they have focused on choice and rights in a way that fails to encompass the full needs of diverse individuals and communities. Reproductive justice reanimates ethical debates about reproductive freedom and shines a light on punitive and misguided practices that historically and currently disproportionately affect the poor, communities of color, and other marginalized peoples.

References

1. Leonard TMB. Laying the foundations for a reproductive justice movement. In Ross LJ, Roberts L, Derkas E, Peoples W, Toure PB, eds., *Radical Reproductive Justice: Foundations, Theory, Practice, Critique*. New York: CUNY Feminist Press; 2017:39–50.
2. Ross LJ. Conceptualizing reproductive justice theory: A manifesto for activism. In Ross LJ, Roberts L, Derkas E, Peoples W, Toure PB, eds., *Radical Reproductive Justice: Foundations, Theory, Practice, Critique*. New York: CUNY Feminist Press; 2017:170–233.
3. Silliman JM, Fried MG, Ross LJ, Gutiérrez E. *Undivided Rights: Women of Color Organizing for Reproductive Justice*, 2nd ed. Chicago: Haymarket Books; 2016.
4. Ross LJ, Solinger R. *Reproductive Justice: An Introduction*. Berkeley: University of California Press; 2017.
5. Ross LJ, Roberts L, Derkas E, Peoples W, Toure PB, eds. *Radical Reproductive Justice: Foundations, Theory, Practice, Critique*. New York: CUNY Feminist Press; 2017.
6. Silliman JM. Introduction. In Bhattacharjee A, Silliman JM, eds., *Policing the National Body: Sex, Race, and Criminalization*. Cambridge, MA: South End Press; 2002:v–xxix.
7. Washington HA. *Medical Apartheid: The Dark History of Medical Experimentation on African Americans*. New York: Doubleday; 2007.

8. Alexandra Minna, S. Sterilized in the name of public health: Race, immigration, and reproductive control in modern California. *Am J Publ Health*. 2005;95(7):1128–38.

9. Lombardo PA. *Three Generations, No Imbeciles: Eugenics, the Supreme Court, and Buck v. Bell*. Baltimore, MD: Johns Hopkins University Press; 2008.

10. Department of Health and Human Services. Consent for sterilization. 2012. https://www.hhs.gov/opa/sites/default/files/consent-for-sterilization-english-updated.pdf

11. Roth R. "If they hand you a paper, you sign it": A call to end the sterilization of women in prison. *Hastings Women's L J*. 2015;26:7.

12. Obstetrics and Gynecology Committee. Committee Opinion No 695 Summary: Sterilization of women: Ethical issues and considerations. *Obstet Gynecol*. 2017;129(4):775–6. https://doi.org/10.1097/AOG.0000000000002013

13. Roberts D. *Killing the Black Body: Race, Reproduction, and The Meaning of Liberty*. New York: Pantheon; 1997.

14. Philadelphia Inquirer Editorial Board. Poverty and Norplant: Can contraception reduce the underclass? *Philadelphia Inquirer*. 1990 Dec 12:18.

15. Native American women uncover Norplant abuses. *Ms*. 1993 Oct;4(2):69.

16. Roberts D. Preface to the Vintage Books edition. In Roberts D, ed., *Killing the Black Body: Race, Reproduction, and the Meaning of Liberty*. New York: Vintage Books; 2017.

17. Louis JM, Menard MK, Gee RE. Racial and ethnic disparities in maternal morbidity and mortality. *Obstet Gynecol*. 2015;125(3):690–4. https://doi.org/10.1097/AOG.0000000000000704

18. Kochanek KD, Murphy SL, Xu J, Tejada-Vera B. Deaths: Final data for 2014 (National Vital Statistics Reports No. Vol. 65, No. 4). CDC. 2016. https://www.cdc.gov/nchs/data/nvsr/nvsr65/nvsr65_04.pdf

19. CDC. Births: Final data for 2015 (National Vital Statistics Reports No. Vol. 66, No. 1). 2017. https://www.cdc.gov/nchs/data/nvsr/nvsr66/nvsr66_01_tables.pdf

20. Contraceptive use in the United States. Guttmacher Institute. 2016 Sep. https://www.guttmacher.org/fact-sheet/contraceptive-use-united-states

21. Characteristics of US abortion patients in 2014 and changes since 2008. Guttmacher Institute. 2016 May. https://www.guttmacher.org/report/characteristics-us-abortion-patients-2014

22. Dehlendorf C, Harris LH, Weitz TA. Disparities in abortion rates: A public health approach. *Am J Publ Health*. 2013;103(10):1772–9.

23. CDC Division of STD Prevention. Sexually transmitted disease surveillance 2016. 2017. https://www.cdc.gov/std/stats16/CDC_2016_STDS_Report-for508WebSep21_2017_1644.pdf

24. Plenty M, Krebs C. Female victims of sexual violence, 1994–2010. Bureau of Justice Statistics. 2013. https://www.bjs.gov/content/pub/pdf/fvsv9410.pdf

25. Lu M, Halfon N. Racial and ethnic disparities in birth outcomes: A life-course perspective. *Matern Child Health J*. 2003;7(1):13–30.

26. Bergin A, Whitaker AK, Terplan M, Gilliam M. Failure to return for intrauterine device insertion after initial clinic visit. *Contraception*. 2009;80(2):217–18. https://doi.org/10.1016/j.contraception.2009.05.088

27. Damm K, Martins S, Gilliam M, Watson S. Postpartum contraceptive use by urban/rural status: An analysis of the Michigan Pregnancy Risk Assessment Monitoring System (PRAMS) data. *Contraception*. 2013;88(3):467. https://doi.org/10.1016/j.contraception.2013.05.139

2

Religiously Affiliated Healthcare Institutions

An Ethical Analysis of What They Mean for Patients, Clinicians, and Our Health System

Lori Freedman PhD and Debra Stulberg MD, MAPP

A high-risk obstetrician recalls an interaction with her laboring patient while explaining that she cannot do her tubal ligation during imminent Cesarean section:

"I went back in the room and I told her that. I said, you know, I can't do your tubal ligation [during the c-section]. And she's like, What are you talking about? My abdomen's going to be wide open, right? I said, Yes. And she said, Well isn't it right there, I mean, isn't it all just right there? Isn't it like kind of easy at that point? And I said, Well yes. She goes, So why can't you? [She] kept looking at me like What are you talking about? So, I sort of had—like I took a deep breath and I thought, Okay, got to start from square one. I said, 'Well this is Saints Hospital (pseudonym). It's a Catholic hospital. I said, Are you aware of any restrictions placed on birth control by the Catholic Church? And she goes, Well . . . I guess I know sort of what you mean, but what does that have to do with me? I'm not Catholic. And you could sort of see it just went on from there. So I told her, you know, that the rule applies to every patient who's within the hospital, that there's certain restrictions placed by Catholic doctrine that mean I can't do this."

Case Background

The patient in this case wants a postpartum tubal ligation and has completed her Medicaid-required consent paperwork for sterilization more than 30 days in advance. She is delivering her third child, suffers from serious health problems that would make another pregnancy dangerous for her, and, due to poverty, already struggles to find transportation from her small town to this Catholic hospital, which is the only hospital within an hour of her home. By policy, Catholic hospitals do not allow tubal ligations or any procedures intended for sterilization. This hospital had been known to allow some exceptions for patients delivering by cesarean section (c-section), but the local bishop had intervened to stop such exceptions in recent years. For this patient, not getting the sterilization procedure she desires will mean she must have a second operation and a second course of anesthesia in order to complete it at a later time. In her case, without intending to, she becomes pregnant again before she is able to have the second surgery.

Ethical Concerns and Questions

The law allows healthcare institutions to restrict care based on religious commitments.[1] How, then, can pregnant patients in need of the restricted care be protected from discrimination and harm? What level of transparency should be required of healthcare facilities with religious restrictions on care, and who should ensure that this information reaches patients long before the crisis point, as occurred in the preceding case? What minimum requirements should be met in exchange for the right to religiously restrict care?

Historical Context of Religious Healthcare

In the United States, more than one hospital bed out of five lies within a religious hospital.[2] The significant market share occupied by religious facilities is an artifact of our peculiar healthcare history. How religion restricts reproductive care within these hospitals is of considerable concern to physicians and poorly understood by patients. Many hospitals, secular and religious, restrict abortion in a variety of circumstances.[2,3] However, Catholic hospitals are particularly notable because they restrict a wider array of services and they constitute 70% of all religious nonprofit hospitals.[4] *The Ethical and Religious Directives for Catholic Healthcare Services*, policies governing care within Catholic facilities, prohibit contraception, sterilization, most fertility treatment, and some forms of miscarriage management, in addition to abortion for any reason.[5]

More than a century ago Catholic and Jewish hospitals were founded by clergy to care for and meet the unique spiritual needs of their relatively marginalized constituents at a time when there was still little medicine could do to cure disease.[6,7] Science advanced during the twentieth century, and medical infrastructure grew, yet the government shied away from developing a cohesive national system as witnessed in other countries such as the United Kingdom. Instead, a patchwork of private, public, academic, and not-for-profit religious and secular hospitals filled needs, city by city.[8] By the late twentieth century, market forces that favored larger systems of managed care provided optimal conditions for Catholic healthcare growth.[6] Members of the Catholic Health Association were well-poised—even encouraged[9]—to share resources when they merged. Nonprofit tax savings aided Catholic health systems in being able to promise needed capital investments when they bought failing hospitals of all types: public, private, religious, and secular.[10]

Fast forward to the current era: Catholic hospital networks have continued to grow, even as other religious hospitals have decreased in number. Widely viewed as charitable institutions deserving of tax breaks and the religious freedom to provide care as they see fit, today Catholic hospitals provide no more Medicaid or charity care than other types of hospitals. Still, US bishops retain control over the care allowed in Catholic hospitals, with decreasing physician discretion and relatively little public awareness. Simultaneously, several Catholic systems have adopted less religious-sounding names. Alexian Brothers' system changed its name to Amita Health, Catholic Healthcare West's system became Dignity Health, and Catholic Health Initiatives system recently merged with Dignity to become the second largest health system in the United States, dubbed CommonSpirit, leaving fewer clues to patients of what to expect inside hospital walls.

Empirical research with physicians and patients about how Catholic doctrine affects ob-gyn care has revealed significant ethical conflicts. Patients are underinformed about the ways in which their physicians' hands are tied when delivering reproductive care,[11,12] and the resulting infringements on patient autonomy and well-being are unequally experienced across the US population.[13,14] Clinicians should understand how religion can constrain care if working in Catholic facilities or if treating patients of reproductive age who have been seen in them.

Catholic Health Doctrine in Practice

To understand what makes Catholic hospitals unique among religiously sponsored hospitals, a good place to start is the *Ethical and Religious Directives for Catholic Healthcare Services*. This document is written by the US Conference of Catholic bishops and enforced at the hospital level by the bishop of the local diocese.[5]

The Directives are not simply guidance. They specifically state: "Catholic health care services must adopt these Directives as policy, require adherence to them within the institution as a condition for medical privileges and employment, and provide appropriate instruction regarding the Directives for administration, medical and nursing staff, and other personnel." The document contains a total of 72 directives, of which 17 govern reproductive care. They prohibit most fertility treatment, surrogate motherhood, all contraception except natural family planning, all sterilization, and abortion in all instances except an emergency.

Postpartum Tubal Sterilization

In relation to tubal ligation and vasectomy, directive 53 states: "Direct sterilization of either men or women, whether permanent or temporary, is not permitted in a Catholic health care institution. Procedures that induce sterility are permitted when their direct effect is the cure or alleviation of a present and serious pathology and a simpler treatment is not available." The second half of this directive leaves room for hospitals to interpret that some tubal ligations are permissible, but interpretations are inconsistent. In some Catholic hospitals, postpartum tubal ligations have been allowed through carve-out agreements (formed prior to 2018)[15] between bishops and doctors, often mediated by lawyers and patient advocates. These can involve the creation of an actual or symbolic non-Catholic operating room within the hospital that is sold to an outside non-Catholic entity and is not beholden to the Directives.

For example, our sample case took place in a hospital with such a carve-out agreement. It was developed after the bishop informed physicians that c-section sterilizations would no longer be permitted (other sterilizations had never been allowed). The agreement permitted physicians from a non-Catholic public health clinic to perform the tubal ligation if they could staff the entire c-section delivery by personnel from their clinic, not the hospital. Physicians were told that if they performed a tubal ligation with hospital-employed staff assisting, the entire agreement could be revoked.

In the case presented, no clinic employee had signed themselves up for the sterilization call team that particular night, and the doctor feared that if she violated protocol and did the tubal ligation anyway, the bishop would follow through on his threat to void their workaround agreement, thereby foreclosing the option for future patients. Thus, despite having a theoretical workaround in place, this patient was unable to receive the tubal ligation she wanted.

In addition to such workaround failures, physicians have reported that workarounds can change with little notice when a new bishop or hospital administration decides to reinterpret the directive and prohibit all sterilizations regardless of circumstance.[16] When a patient is delivering by c-section and wants a tubal ligation, the option of referring her to another facility for the sterilization means subjecting her to a second surgery at a later time. This risk is described by many ob-gyns as ethically unacceptable.

In other cases, ob-gyns describe referral for a later tubal ligation as effectively impossible for other reasons. For example, the patient's insurance may only be accepted by the Catholic hospital due to her employer- or government-based plan. Or, the patient may lose her insurance shortly after the end of her pregnancy and return later for her desired sterilization with no means to cover the cost. In these circumstances, performing the desired sterilization during the delivery hospitalization is the only feasible means for the patient to receive the family planning method she desires, yet the Catholic hospital makes it impossible. Qualitative and historical research, as well as guidelines published by Catholic healthcare leadership, indicate a broad trend of narrowing of exceptions to the sterilization prohibition.[6,17,18]

Miscarriage and Other Pregnancy Complications

Abortion is also prohibited, and the Directives make critical distinctions between direct and indirect abortion that have implications for miscarriage management and a wider array of obstetric complications.[19] Directive 45 begins: "Abortion (that is, the directly intended termination of pregnancy before viability or the directly intended destruction of a viable fetus) is never permitted. Every procedure whose sole immediate effect is the termination of pregnancy before viability is an abortion, which, in its moral context, includes the interval between conception and implantation of the embryo."

But two directives discuss the permissibility of what the authors call "indirect abortion." First, with regard to ectopic pregnancy, directive 48 states: "In case of extrauterine pregnancy, no intervention is morally licit which constitutes a direct abortion." No specific guidance is given on whether or in what circumstances methotrexate constitutes a direct abortion. In relation to obstetric complications in general, directive 47 says more about the concept of indirect abortion and when it is allowed. It says: "Operations, treatments, and medications that have as their direct purpose the cure of a proportionately serious pathological condition of a pregnant woman are permitted when they cannot be safely postponed until the unborn child is viable, even if they will result in the death of the unborn child."

Directives 48 and 47 show that the distinction between *direct versus indirect* is of more theological than medical significance. Catholic teaching has long been guided by the Principle of Double Effect, which holds that when an action is expected to have two effects—one good and one bad—the decision about whether to proceed with the action should be based on the intended good effect, even if the bad one is a foreseeable "side effect" of the process. Under this principle, if the clinician causes the abortion in the process of trying to do something else, then the intent is not abortion (indirect).[20] That is, if the physician removes a cancerous uterus or treats chorioamniotis by emptying the uterus, and, in the process the fetus dies, this may be permissible per the Directives. But the physician cannot perform an abortion with the intent to do so in itself. As such, some abortions do happen in Catholic hospitals, technically speaking, but they must only occur in the process of treating very specific medical emergencies, usually with the preapproval of the Catholic hospital ethics committee charged with interpreting and applying the Directives.

Medical Professional Guidelines

Major physician bodies have produced guidelines asserting that physicians' freedom to refuse care based on conscience is not unlimited. The American College of Obstetricians and Gynecologists (ACOG) committee on ethics issued a statement which concludes: "Any conscientious refusal that conflicts with a patient's well-being should be accommodated only if the primary duty to the patient can be fulfilled."[21] The American Medical Association (AMA) code of ethics specifies that refusals are not acceptable when risk of harm or delay "would significantly adversely affect the patient's physical or emotional well-being; and when the patient is not reasonably able to access needed treatment from another qualified physician." However, these professional guidelines say little to address institutionally enforced refusals that override physician conscience. And since 39% of reproductive-age women in the United States live in a county where Catholic hospitals have a high or dominant market share,[22] many patients are not reasonably able to access treatment at a non-Catholic facility.

Physician Experiences and Concerns

Ob-gyns working in Catholic hospitals have concerns about how religion affects patient care. Most ob-gyn residents trained in religious facilities intend to provide full-scope reproductive care, but compared to their peers in nonreligious residencies, they feel less satisfied with their family planning training and less confident in their skills to provide common reproductive procedures such as insertion of contraceptive devices and manual vacuum aspiration.[23] In 2011, a national physician survey asked those ob-gyns whose primary workplace was religiously affiliated "Have you ever experienced conflict with your hospital over its religious policies for patient care?" Responses showed that 52% of ob-gyns working in a Catholic facility said yes; for comparison, at Christian (non-Catholic) hospitals 17% said yes, and at Jewish hospitals 9% said yes they had experienced this kind of conflict.

In a subsequent qualitative study from which this chapter's case was drawn, interviews with a subset of Catholic hospital ob-gyns revealed specific scenarios of concern beyond sterilization. While many physicians accepted that certain typically outpatient services were not allowed, such as contraception, early/uncomplicated abortion, infertility services, and interval sterilizations, restrictions that impacted inpatient care were of considerable concern to the physicians, and some expressed serious moral distress.[17,19,24]

Physician offered many scenarios in which pregnant women presented with serious pregnancy complications and Catholic hospital policy prevented them from providing standard counseling and treatment.[19,24,25] Women whose stories have been reported publicly, such as Tamesha Means and Mindy Swank, described their experiences of being repeatedly turned away from Catholic hospitals during miscarriage, enduring pain, infection, and extended emotional suffering as a result.[26] In cases like those of

Means, Swank, and even Savita Halappanavar in Ireland, who died as a result in 2011 and whose case catalyzed legal reform there,[27,28] when a patient's membranes rupture (commonly known as her "water breaking") well before the fetus is viable, there is a risk to the woman of a serious infection setting in. At the same time, a fetus remote from viability has little to no likelihood of surviving to viability with the membranes ruptured, so physicians in many circumstances see this as a certain miscarriage. In most non-Catholic hospitals, the patient would be offered the option to watch and wait as long as she does not develop signs of infection, as well as the option to induce labor with medications or possibly have a dilation and evacuation (D&E) procedure. The medication and procedural treatments are intended to expedite delivery or removal of the pre-viable fetus to prevent infection from developing and to help speed the completion of a process that started on its own so the woman can begin recovery sooner. Women's preferences for miscarriage treatment are complex, but research has shown that offering all options and engaging in shared decision-making leads to the greatest patient satisfaction, and patients who receive their preferred treatment report better mental health and quality of life after.[29] However, physicians in many Catholic hospitals say their hands are tied unless and until the woman starts to show signs of infection. These restrictions are likely to affect many patients: in a national survey of reproductive-age women, 31% reported they had ever received care for a pregnancy complication, miscarriage, or loss.[12,30]

In research about these scenarios, ob-gyns discussed treatment options that they saw as important or necessary for preserving the woman's health or life, while the Catholic hospitals where they worked defined the treatment as a prohibited abortion. What qualifies as an *indirect abortion* (that can be performed in some circumstances under Catholic teaching) varies in different reporting from different Catholic hospitals. Physicians working in Catholic hospitals are thus left to rely on local interpretation of the Directives. In some cases, they can or must petition their hospital's ethics committee when they think such a treatment is needed and await a ruling about whether or not they can treat patients in accordance with medical standards.

Referrals for Abortion

While many ob-gyns describe their Catholic hospitals allowing them to refer patients for most or all services that are prohibited under the Directives, abortion is sometimes the exception.[31-33] Some physicians face pressure to make these referrals in a hidden or limited fashion, if they can make them at all. Some describe receiving none of the common administrative or nursing support they usually receive for referrals—such as faxing medical records or assisting with appointment scheduling—when the needed service is an abortion and the setting is Catholic. This differentiation between abortion and other prohibited services, such as sterilization or reversible contraception, can exacerbate the existing shame and stigma that patients face when seeking abortion.

Patient Awareness and Preferences

While institutional religious restrictions on care are distressing to many physicians who work under them, it is difficult to discern patients' understanding of the issue. However, studies have begun to show that women lack sufficient knowledge to make informed decisions about where to seek care. A national survey of women of reproductive age shows that 37% of women whose primary ob-gyn hospital is Catholic do not know that it is Catholic, and, within this subset, about two-thirds believe it to be secular and the other third believes it is affiliated with another religion.[30] Low-income women attending a Catholic hospital are significantly less likely to correctly identify its religion than women with higher household incomes. Furthermore, even women who know a hospital is Catholic appear unable to anticipate how specifically care is restricted within Catholic hospitals. Two vignette-based studies showed that many women randomized to fictitious hospitals named "St. Ignatius" and "St. John's" expected to be able to get sterilization, contraception, and miscarriage management needs met.[11,34]

What's clear is that women want to know about restrictions on their care. When the aforementioned national survey asked women if they thought it was important to know if a hospital had a religious affiliation, only 34.5% said they felt it was somewhat or very important.[35] However, when followed up with a statement informing women that some hospitals restrict some ob-gyn care for religious reasons, women became more curious. In response to the next question, "How important is it for you to know what care is restricted?," the vast majority (80.7%) of women found it important to know. This discrepancy indicates that the idea that care can be restricted for religious reasons may be a new one.

Indeed, preliminary qualitative research on the topic indicates exactly that.[36] One transgender man was stunned to have his hysterectomy abruptly canceled because hospital clergy equated it to a prohibited sterilization. He did not even recognize that it was a Catholic hospital initially, "I didn't think about the whole religious aspect of it. I had no idea. It kind of just dawned on me when [the doctor] called me to let me know that the nuns at the hospital had rejected my procedure." In different case, a woman who went to a Catholic hospital in need of an abortion was surprised to be turned away; it was the only source of care in her area for indigent patients. She explained that she thought the religion was meant to be more comforting than proscriptive, "Sometimes they just use [religion] because they're hospitals, of course, you know, so they want people to feel safe." A third patient, who was raised Catholic, was surprised when she was unable to schedule a tubal ligation in her Catholic hospital. She reflected on her dismay, "I grew up in that faith, so it was just like a connection for me. You know what I mean? I figured a tubal ligation, that's not terminating a pregnancy. It's nothing to be frowned upon. Surprise to me, it was." Patients prefer transparency and options, and mounting research reveals that the public face of Catholic facilities, reflected by websites and hospital names, do little to help patient anticipate or avoid the difficult experiences of being refused care.[35-37]

Bioethical Issues

Patient autonomy, and patients' related freedom from religious restrictions on care, are at risk when healthcare facilities are owned and governed by religious organizations. Religious freedom is highly valued in the United States and in many countries across the globe. The legal and ethical framework to protect healthcare providers from having to provide services that conflict with their religious beliefs is well established and vigorously defended, but the rights of patients to receive lawful medical care motivated by their own beliefs and values deserves equally vehement protection.[38] Patients often lack appropriate information and meaningful alternatives. We have shown that many women do not know how religion will affect their care until they have already been delayed, denied, or worse. Denials of care can compound the stigma that patients already feel when accessing sexual and reproductive healthcare. Some patients, even if informed about religious restrictions, do not live in areas with—or have insurance that allows for—a choice of providers.

In the case of Catholic healthcare, the religious freedom is concentrated within the hands of Church leadership, not the employees or patients of Catholic hospitals. As we have shown here, many clinicians do not support the way that religious restrictions affect care. Some experience it as substandard, coercive, and deceitful. While in theory providers can simply choose to work elsewhere, choices may be limited by geography and degree of healthcare market saturation by religious entities. In some states, nearly half of the hospital beds are in Catholic facilities.

An additional ethical consideration is how religious restrictions on care disproportionately impact vulnerable women. Nationwide, 53% of births in Catholic hospitals are to women of color (compared to 49% in non-Catholic hospitals), and in some states this disproportionate impact is especially dramatic; for example, 80% of New Jersey Catholic hospital births are to women of color, compared to 53% in non-Catholic hospitals.[14] The facts that women of color are more likely to give birth in Catholic hospitals and that having a higher income is associated with greater likelihood of correctly identifying one's hospital as Catholic[39] point to a structural problem and a deeper injustice that compounds existing racial and economic disparities in health.

Hospitals are a limited resource, heavily regulated by governing bodies. Thus, if a religious hospital is seen as already meeting most community needs, another hospital will not be built. At a systemic level, vulnerable women's reproductive healthcare has been sacrificed time and again as Catholic health systems expand with support from municipalities, states, and federal grants.[40] Given that religious hospitals occupy a sizable share of the healthcare market while prohibiting some of the most common, safe, and desired reproductive services, fiduciary and professional obligations toward patients must be rigorously assessed. Few, if any, other areas of healthcare proliferate with religious constraints on common and critical care that create systemically reproduced practices of inferior treatment.

Implications for Clinicians

Healthcare professionals have a fiduciary duty to insist that all people's healthcare needs are met at the standard of care, regardless of where the patient seeks care. When legal solutions to injustice and inequity in healthcare

are absent, the medical profession can and often does work to address them through guidelines, accreditation, and evidence-based recommendations. Thus we propose that clinicians working with pregnant patients, including nurse practitioners, physician assistants, certified nurse midwives, and physicians within family medicine, ob-gyn, maternal-fetal medicine, and internal medicine, hold themselves and their colleagues accountable to ensure optimal pathways to care.

To do this, these clinicians should

1. Consider the implications carefully before working in a religious system.
2. For outpatient care, give potential new patients full information about how services are limited by religious ownership or affiliation and engage in an informed decision-making process about whether this is the right medical practice to meet her needs. Ensure that limitations are clear and accessible on websites.
3. Develop strong pathways to needed care—including referrals—for abortion at each stage, miscarriage management, and postpartum plans for sterilization and contraception. Respect patients' preferences and work to see these are carried out.
4. Maintain privileges in nonreligious hospitals, and, if not possible, maintain trusted relationships with colleagues who can care for patients, offer the full range of options (e.g., if the patient wants a postpartum sterilization or long-acting reversible contraceptive), and make plans for transfer of care even when it means lost income.
5. Discuss where to seek miscarriage management with all prenatal patients. Find out who is best suited to provide all options and high-quality treatment and make sure all staff members know about this. Counsel patients honestly about what to expect if they present to a hospital with religious restrictions on care.
6. Develop phone triage for active miscarriage—with special concern for women in their second trimester. Do not assume institutions will take this on. Communicate clearly with nurses and other staff members about the implications of care to avoid confusion. If nurses (or other staff responding to emergency calls) are employees of an institution that restricts what they can tell patients, consider contracting with an outside service for unbiased phone counseling.

We recognize that it is not in the physician's own professional interest to dissuade a patient from coming to her or his medical practice, or to engage superiors in difficult conversations about how to protect patients from religious restrictions. However, we believe many Catholic hospital physicians we interviewed would find their consciences relieved and moral distress diminished by knowing that patients had fully considered what it means to be cared for under religious rules. While policy safeguards on the institutional religious freedom to restrict healthcare have yet to materialize, more can be done at the professional level to improve transparency, autonomy, and justice for patients.

References

1. Lynch HF, Cohen IG, Sepper E. *Law, Religion, and Health in the United States*. New York: Cambridge University Press; 2017.
2. Hasselbacher LA, Hebert LE, Liu Y, Stulberg DB. "My hands are tied": Abortion restrictions and providers' experiences in religious and nonreligious health care systems. *Perspect Sex Reprod Health* 2020;52(2):107–115.
3. Zeldovich VB, Rocca CH, Langton C, Landy U, Ly ES, Freedman LR. Abortion policies in US teaching hospitals: Formal and informal parameters beyond the law. *Obstet Gynecol.* 2020;135:1296–1305.
4. Uttley L, Khaikin C, Hasbrouck P. Growth of Catholic hospitals and health systems: 2016 update of the miscarriage of medicine report. MergerWatch; 2016. http://static1.1.sqspcdn.com/static/f/816571/27061007/1465224862580/MW_Update-2016-MiscarrOfMedicine-report.pdf
5. US Conference of Catholic Bishops. *The Ethical and Religious Directives for Catholic Healthcare Services*. Washington DC: United States Conference of Catholic Bishops; 2018.
6. Wall BM. *American Catholic Hospitals: A Century of Changing Markets and Missions*. New Brunswick, NJ: Rutgers University Press; 2011.
7. Joyce KM. The evil of abortion and the greater good of the faith: Negotiating Catholic survival in the twentieth-century American health care system. *Religion American Culture*. 2002;12:91–121.
8. Starr P. *The Social Transformation of American Medicine*. New York: Basic Books; 1982.
9. Nygren DJ. Troubled waters: Remaining a beacon amid change. *Health Prog.* 2013;94.
10. Young GJ, Chou C-H, Alexander J, Lee S-YD, Raver E. Provision of community benefits by tax-exempt US hospitals. *N Engl J Med.* 2013;368:1519–27.
11. Guiahi M, Sheeder J, Teal S. Are women aware of religious restrictions on reproductive health at Catholic hospitals? A survey of women's expectations and preferences for family planning care. *Contraception.* 2014;90:429–34.
12. Freedman LR, Hebert LE, Battistelli MF, Stulberg DB. Religious hospital policies on reproductive care: What do patients want to know? *Am J Obstet Gynecol.* 2018;218:251. e1–e9.

13. Hill EL, Slusky D, Ginther D. *Medically Necessary but Forbidden: Reproductive Health Care in Catholic-Owned Hospitals.* Cambridge, MA: National Bureau of Economic Research; 2017.
14. Shepherd K, Reiner Platt E, Franke K, Boylen E. *Bearing Faith: The Limits of Catholic Health Care for Women of Color.* New York: Columbia Law School; 2018 Jan 19.
15. Meyer H. New Catholic directives could complicate mergers and partnerships. Modern Healthcare. 2018. https://www.modernhealthcare.com/article/20180719/NEWS/180719880/
16. Freedman L. Yes, the church should be liable when doctrines interfere with safe medical care for women: New research into medical decisions at church-run facilities. The New Republic. 2014 Jan 1. https://newrepublic.com/article/116034/catholic-hospitals-lawsuit-usccb-doctrines-determine-care
17. Stulberg DB, Hoffman Y, Dahlquist IH, Freedman LR. Tubal ligation in Catholic hospitals: A qualitative study of ob-gyns' experiences. *Contraception* 2014;90:422–8.
18. Panicola M, Hamel R. Catholic Identity and the Reshaping of Health Care. 2015. Health Progress: Journal of the Catholic Health Association of the United States. Sept-Oct 2015, 46–56. https://www.chausa.org/publications/health-progress/article/september-october-2015/catholic-identity-and-the-reshaping-of-health-care
19. Freedman LR, Stulberg DB. Conflicts in care for obstetric complications in Catholic hospitals. *AJOB Primary Res.* 2013;4:1–10.
20. Markwell HJ, Brown BF. Bioethics for clinicians: 27. Catholic bioethics. *Can Med Assoc J.* 2001;165:189–92.
21. ACOG Committee. Opinion No. 385 November 2007: The limits of conscientious refusal in reproductive medicine. *Obstet Gynecol.* 2007;110:1203–8.
22. Drake C, Jarlenski M, Zhang Y, Polsky D. Market share of US Catholic hospitals and associated geographic network access to reproductive health services. *JAMA Network Open.* 2020;3:e1920053-e.
23. Guiahi M, Hoover J, Swartz M, Teal S. Impact of Catholic hospital affiliation during obstetrics and gynecology residency on the provision of family planning. *J Grad Med Educ.* 2017;9:440–6.
24. Freedman LR, Landy U, Steinauer J. When there's a heartbeat: Miscarriage management in Catholic-owned hospitals. *Am J Public Health.* 2008;98:1774–8.
25. ACOG. Prelabor rupture of membranes: ACOG Practice Bulletin, Number 217. *Obstet Gynecol.* 2020;135:e80–e97.
26. Kaye J, Amiri B, Melling L, Dalven J. Health care denied: Patients and physicians speak out about Catholic hospitals and the threat to women's health and lives. American Civil Liberties Union; 2016. https://www.aclu.org/issues/reproductive-freedom/religion-and-reproductive-rights/health-care-denied
27. Berer M. Termination of pregnancy as emergency obstetric care: The interpretation of Catholic health policy and the consequences for pregnant women: An analysis of the death of Savita Halappanavar in Ireland and similar cases. *Reprod Health Matters.* 2013;21:9–17.
28. O'Connor A. How the death of Savita Halappanavar changed the abortion debate. The *Irish Examiner.* 2017 Oct 28.
29. Wallace RR, Goodman S, Freedman LR, Dalton VK, Harris LH. Counseling women with early pregnancy failure: Utilizing evidence, preserving preference. *Patient Educ Counsel.* 2010;81:454–61.

30. Wascher J, Freedman L, Hebert L, Stulberg D. Do women know whether their hospital is Catholic? Results from a national survey. *Contraception.* 2018;98(6):498–503.
31. Stulberg DB, Jackson RA, Freedman LR. Referrals for services prohibited in Catholic health care facilities. *Perspect Sex Reprod Health.* 2016;48:111–17.
32. Kaunitz AM, Benrubi GI, Barbieri RL, et al. Ethics and referral for abortion. *Am J Obstet Gynecol.* 2009;200:e9; author reply e-10.
33. The National Catholic Bioethics Center (NCBC). Statements by NCBC Ethicsists, May 1, 2015. Transfer of Care vs. Referral: A Crucial Moral Distinction. https://www.ncbcenter.org/resources-and-statements-cms/transfer-of-care-vs-referral-a-crucial-moral-distinction
34. Stulberg DB, Guiahi M, Hebert LE, Freedman LR. Women's expectation of receiving reproductive health care at catholic and non-catholic hospitals. *Perspect Sex Reprod Health.* 2019 Sep;51(3):135–42. doi:10.1363/psrh.12118.
35. Freedman LR, Hebert L, Battistelli M, Stulberg DB. Religious hospital policies on reproductive care: What do patients want to know? *Am J Obstet Gynecol.* 2018 Feb;218(2):251.e1–251.e9.
36. Freedman L. Women's perspectives on receiving care in religiously affiliated institutions. MacLean Center for Bioethics, Reproductive Ethics Lecture Series, University of Chicago; 2017.
37. Guiahi M, Teal SB, Swartz M, Huynh S, Schiller G, Sheeder J. What are women told when requesting family planning services at clinics associated with Catholic hospitals? A mystery caller study. *Perspect Sex Reprod Health.* 2017;49(4):207–12.
38. Sepper E. Taking conscience seriously. *VA Law Rev.* 2012:1501–75.
39. Wascher JM, Hebert LE, Freedman LR, Stulberg DB. Do women know whether their hospital is Catholic? Results from a national survey. *Contraception.* 2018;98:498–503.
40. Dardick H. Aldermen approve $5.6M subsidy for Presence Health despite flap over abortion services, birth control. *Chicago Tribune.* 2018 Jan 12.

3

Contemporary Challenges to Providing Confidential Reproductive Healthcare to Minors

Amber Truehart MD, MSc, Lee Hasselbacher JD,
and Julie Chor MD, MPH

Nina Jones is 16 years old when she comes to Dr. Smith with her maternal grandmother for her first gynecologic visit. In the initial interview, Nina tells Dr. Smith that she has been sexually active for several months and that she scheduled her appointment to discuss her contraceptive options. She and her current partner have been using condoms intermittently. Nina lives with her mother and younger sister but looks to her maternal grandmother, who she asked to be present with her during this appointment, for advice about personal issues such as sex. She has not discussed her sexual activity with her mother, who told Nina years ago that she did not want her to have sex until marriage. Her mother told her that she became pregnant with Nina when she was only 15 and that she did not want the same thing to happen to Nina. Since Nina was considering an intrauterine device, she was asked for and agreed to provide a urine sample to test for pregnancy and sexually transmitted infections. The pregnancy test came back positive. Dr. Smith asked Nina's grandmother to step out of the exam room before discussing these results with Nina, stating that it is her standard practice to ask family members to step out of the room during visits to allow patients the opportunity to ask questions that may be embarrassing to ask in front of family. Dr. Smith shared the results with Nina, who was upset and overwhelmed. Nina explained to Dr. Smith that she did not want to tell her mother about this yet and asked Dr. Smith about her pregnancy options. Dr. Smith asked Nina if she wanted her grandmother to return to the room and Nina agreed. Nina, Nina's grandmother, and Dr. Smith proceeded with pregnancy options counseling, and Nina left with the plan to return in 2 weeks to discuss her plans further with Dr. Smith. Nina also tested positive for a sexually transmitted infection, and Dr. Smith sent in an electronic prescription for an antibiotic. Later that day, Nina's mother, Mrs. Jones, received a phone call from their pharmacy stating that her daughter's prescription for her antibiotic was ready. Not knowing what this prescription was for, Mrs. Jones opened Nina's electronic medical record and found "pregnancy" and "sexually transmitted disease testing" included under Nina's list of medical conditions. Mrs. Jones calls Dr. Smith and angrily confronts her, stating that she should have been asked permission for Nina to see a gynecologist and that Dr. Smith should have called to tell her that her daughter is pregnant.

Questions for Consideration

1. How can providers navigate confidentiality obligations with minor patients?
2. How can providers navigate conflicts with a minor patient's parent?
3. What must providers consider in order to protect a minor patient's confidentiality?
4. How can providers improve systems and structures to support confidential care for a minor patient?

Minors in many states have a legal right to consent for reproductive health services, including contraception, pregnancy care, sexually transmitted infection testing and treatment, and (to varying degrees) abortion care. A patient's right to consent is usually paired with a right to confidentiality. However, as this case illustrates, clinicians treating minors can encounter numerous challenges to ensuring these patients' confidentiality. Laws establishing the right to consent for minors recognize that some minors may not seek certain health services if they were forced to involve a parent. Prior research has shown that youth may forego needed healthcare due to concerns about privacy and confidentiality, and these concerns are linked to lower use of contraceptives and higher adolescent pregnancy rates.[1-3] While many minors do involve a parent when seeking reproductive health, preserving confidentiality and helping a young person navigate their own circumstances can build trust within the patient–provider relationship and improve health outcomes for young people.

To help healthcare providers anticipate and navigate these challenges, this chapter starts with a review of policies and laws that impact consent and confidentiality for minors seeking reproductive healthcare services. We go on to discuss the public health origins of minor consent and confidentiality laws and the research that informs our understanding of how adolescents and healthcare providers engage on these issues. We then explore the relationship between these laws, a provider's ethical obligations, and the concept of adolescent autonomy. Finally, we consider how the infrastructure of contemporary medical practice can undermine the legal protections afforded to minors, specifically focusing on electronic medical records, electronic prescriptions, and dependent insurance. In addressing the questions posed earlier, we will advise providers how to optimize their minor patients' ability to access needed services while maintaining a trusting patient–provider relationship.

Legal Framework for Consent and Confidentiality in Adolescent Reproductive Healthcare

Consent

Adolescent minors who have not reached the "age of majority" (18 in most states) typically need parental consent for medical care. However, some federal and state laws grant minors the ability to consent to health services independently. These are often state laws based either on the *status* of the minor or the *services* the minor requests.[6,7] Status laws authorize certain categories of minors—those who are married, emancipated, or a certain age—to consent to all of their own medical care. Service laws allow every minor to consent when they are seeking a particular service, such as contraception, testing and treatment for sexually transmitted infections, pregnancy-related care, or HIV/AIDS care.[4,6] In 1977, the US Supreme Court ruled that the constitutional right to privacy applies to minors' reproductive decisions, including a minor's access to contraceptive services and abortion care.[4,8,9] Courts have rejected laws requiring parental consent for contraception, but the US Supreme Court has allowed laws requiring parental consent or parental notification before a minor has an abortion as long as there is an alternate path—such as judicial waiver—for a young person who feels they cannot involve their parents to access abortion care.[6,10] Every state has at least one law granting capacity to consent based on either the status of a young person or the services sought. The age at which these laws apply vary from state to state, but many laws apply to individuals aged 12 or 14 and older.[6]

The "mature minor doctrine" also establishes a framework for minors to consent to mainstream medical care when it entails minimal risk, is provided non-negligently, the minor demonstrates maturity and decision-making capacity, and consent is voluntary.[4,10] Providers should review their state's laws. If a state law does not create an explicit right to consent, in some states health providers may rely on the mature minor doctrine, along with the constitutional right to privacy, as justification for accepting the consent of mature minors seeking reproductive health services.[11] In addition, parents can still provide consent for care but waive their right to health information or disclosure by agreeing to confidentiality for the minor and their provider. Providers can offer forms for parents to sign that would establish this confidentiality agreement. Conversely, in cases where they determine a minor lacks the maturity or decision-making capacity, providers are neither legally nor ethically obligated to allow the minor to consent for care.

Confidentiality

Minors' legal ability to consent to reproductive healthcare does not necessarily guarantee confidential treatment. Rules defining the boundaries of confidential healthcare for a minor can be found in federal and state laws, regulations, and professional practice guidelines. Confidentiality can also be affected by individual clinic and insurance practices.

In many states, minor consent laws contain language addressing confidentiality; for example, some laws specify that when a minor has consented to care, information about that care cannot be shared without permission.[4] Other types of laws (e.g., child abuse and neglect and medical privacy laws) also specify when disclosure is required, permitted, or prohibited.

The Health Insurance Portability and Accountability Act (HIPAA) Privacy Rule requires healthcare providers and insurers to protect confidential health information, but state laws governing parental access to minor health records can render this protection moot. In certain circumstances the minor may have the same privacy rights as an adult, such as when the minor has the legal right to consent to or receive care or when a parent has assented to an agreement of confidentiality between the minor and provider.[9]

However, even in those cases under HIPAA, parents or guardians may access a minor's protected health information. Note that states can give citizens more protections, so if state or other laws explicitly regulate disclosure of information to a parent, those laws are controlling rather than the HIPAA Privacy Rule.[9–10,12]

When state laws do not provide any guidance on whether disclosure is permitted or prohibited, healthcare providers have discretion about whether and what to communicate with a parent, even in situations where the minor is able to consent to care on their own.[9] Under HIPAA, if any patient clearly states that disclosure could endanger him or her, providers must accommodate their request to send communications by alternative means or to alternative locations, and health plans are required to accommodate such requests if reasonable.[13]

There are also state laws which may require breaches of confidentiality. Providers may be required to make public health reports of communicable diseases, which include sexually transmitted infections, for further investigation. Such reporting may not be anonymous, as communicable disease reporting laws often require that personal information be disclosed to governmental agencies. While parents are not necessarily notified, depending on state laws, providers may choose to disclose results to parents. Mandatory reporting laws require healthcare professionals to breach confidentiality in order to report suspicions of child abuse and neglect, including sexual abuse. Providers may also be required to disclose in situations where a minor is presenting a serious risk of harm to self, including suicidal ideation or homicidal threats.[14,15]

Certain federal programs, including Medicaid and the Title X Family Planning Program, protect the confidentiality of reproductive health services. Medicaid provides health insurance coverage for low-income individuals, including coverage for "family planning services." Medicaid rules require confidential family planning services be made available to sexually active minors of childbearing age who desire them and are eligible for the program.[16–18] Title X is a federal grant program designed to provide access to contraceptive services, supplies, and information to all who want and need them, with a focus on serving low-income individuals. Title X guidelines specify that clinics receiving funding must provide family planning services without regard to age and that services must be confidential.[4,16,19] Courts have invalidated mandates that would require parental consent or disclosure to parents when minors receive family planning services through Medicaid and Title X.[9,20]

Public Health Framework Supporting Consent and Confidentiality in Adolescent Reproductive Healthcare

A public health framework that promotes and protects the health of individuals and their communities provided the impetus for laws giving adolescents the ability to consent for reproductive healthcare and to obtain this care confidentially. The principal concern underlying these laws was not whether or not a minor had the *right* to consent or the *right* to confidential healthcare. Instead, these laws were a response to social shifts in the 1970s that many associated with a rise in pregnancy rates among unmarried adolescents. These social changes included a rise in the average age of marriage, an increase in the proportion of adolescents who were sexually active,[21] expanded access to contraception primarily through new family planning clinic programs,[22] a decrease in social pressure for pregnant adolescents to marry, and the legalization of abortion.[23] During this same time period, epidemiologic data started to reveal that adolescent pregnancy was associated with poorer health outcomes for both young women and their infants.[24] The public health objectives of laws permitting minors to consent for reproductive health services were to help adolescent girls avoid pregnancy, optimize care when pregnant, and prevent and treat sexually transmitted infections.

Today, nearly one in eight adolescents under the age of 15 has been sexually active,[25] and adolescents continue to disproportionately face adverse reproductive health outcomes. Sexually active adolescents and young adults aged 15–24 years account for half of all new sexually transmitted infections diagnoses, and those aged 13–24 years account for nearly a quarter of new HIV diagnoses.[26] While teen pregnancies peaked in the 1990s, they have steadily declined since.[27,28] Between 2008 and 2013, the pregnancy rate among girls aged 15–19 years declined substantially (from 68 to 43 per 1,000 women and girls 15–19 years of age).[28] Declines in adolescent pregnancy and unintended pregnancy rates are largely attributed to more frequent use of contraception and use of more effective methods of contraception.[28] Contemporary data, therefore, underscore the persistent need to ensure adolescents' access to such reproductive health services.

Research supports the public health position that confidentiality of care plays an integral role in whether adolescents will actually use the reproductive health services they are allowed to access without parental consent. One study found that 47% of adolescents reported they would stop using all sexual healthcare services if their parents were notified they were seeking contraception.[29] Additional adolescents in this study indicated that they would discontinue some services or delay testing or treatment of sexually transmitted infections if their parents were notified that they were seeking this care.[29] Adolescents also commonly report concerns for confidentiality as a reason for not seeking medical care.[30] Ford et al. found that 18.7% of adolescents reported foregoing medical care in the past year due to concerns about confidentiality, especially among adolescents who were daily smokers, frequently used alcohol, or were sexually active.[30] A study using data from the 2013–2015 National Survey of Family Growth found that 15- to 17-year-olds who were covered under Medicaid were less likely to express concerns about confidentiality compared to their peers covered under their parents' private insurance (adjusted risk ratio = 0.61; confidence interval, 0.41–0.91).[31] Furthermore, this study found that concerns about confidentiality were associated with a decreased likelihood of obtaining contraceptive care in the past year among sexually experienced girls and women.[31] The existing data support the conclusion that without confidentiality, many teenagers would be unwilling to seek important medical information or access care. Higher risk groups who engage in smoking, alcohol use, or sexual activity may be especially vulnerable to not seeking care due to confidentiality.

Based on the preceding body of research, professional medical organizations such as the American Medical Association (AMA), the American College of Obstetricians and Gynecologists (ACOG), American Academy of Family Physicians (AAFP), and Society for Adolescent Medicine (SAM) have recognized the importance of adolescent confidentiality and have all issued official statements advocating that confidential reproductive health services should be available to minors[32-36] and were integral in supporting consent laws. These organizations recommend that adolescent reproductive healthcare providers discuss confidentiality at the initial visit three times: with the adolescent alone, with parents or caregivers alone (if present), and with both the adolescent and parents/caregivers together.[32-36] Specifically, providers are encouraged to discuss what topics and services are or are not confidential. They also suggest that adolescent patients should be informed about situations or circumstances where they would not be guaranteed confidentiality.

Ethical Framework Supporting Consent and Confidentiality in Adolescent Reproductive Healthcare

The most common ethical framework in American medicine is principlism, which analyzes questions of healthcare ethics through four principles: nonmaleficence, beneficence, justice, and respect for autonomy.[37] The principles of beneficence and nonmaleficence are foundational to the public health arguments behind laws that permit adolescent minors to consent to confidential reproductive health services. These laws allow healthcare providers to act beneficently toward their minor patients through the provision of safe, medically appropriate care that some minor patients would not seek were they required to obtain parental consent. Furthermore, divulging information to parents about their adolescent's sexual and reproductive health may lead to potentially harmful medical and social consequences for some patients. Therefore, by allowing clinicians to maintain adolescent patients' desired confidentiality about issues of sexual and reproductive health, providers are able to adhere to the principle of nonmaleficence and avoid putting some patients at risk of the harms of undesired disclosure of sensitive information.

Laws pertaining to adolescent minors' right to confidentiality and/or consent for reproductive health procedures also adhere to the principle of justice.[37] Specifically, these laws adhere to egalitarian theories of justice in that they apply to minors regardless of socioeconomic status, race/ethnicity, or other demographic or social factors. While this aspect of these laws cannot ensure that providers will in fact do so, the universality of these laws ensures that providers are able to offer all minors the same considerations in decision-making.

Principlism also requires consideration of the autonomy of both adolescents and their parents. *Autonomy* is defined as "self-rule that is free from both controlling interference by others and limitations that prevent meaningful choice, such as inadequate understanding."[37] Intimately tied to the concept of autonomy and autonomous decision-making is the concept of decision-making capacity. With adults, competence is a *legal* determination regarding whether an individual has the legal right to make a decision, and an individual can only be deemed incompetent by a judge.[38] Minors are defined by law to be incompetent, rendering them unable to, for example, sign legal agreements such as contracts. Decisional capacity, however, is a *clinical* determination, defined as an individual's ability to make a decision based on his or her ability to understand key information, medical circumstances and consequences, to consider available treatment options, and to express a choice.[38]

As previously discussed, adolescent minors ordinarily require parental consent for medical care outside of specific services and situations, thus limiting their autonomy. Pediatric care generally involves a therapeutic triad of provider-parent-patient, with the parent(s) largely assuming responsibility for medical decision-making. Parents are presumed to act in accordance with their children's best interest and to advocate for their children's values and preferences.[39,40] Arguments in favor of deferring most decision-making to parents include concerns over the difficulty of determining whether minors have achieved decision-making capacity.[39,40] Further argument in favor of delaying a minors' decision-making is that such a delay allows minors the time to obtain the life experiences and knowledge needed to eventually assume decision-making capacity.[39,40] Additionally, while some neuroscience research has found that the brains of most 12-year-olds have developed structurally to allow for decision-making capacity, the early development of the brain's reward system versus the late development of the brain's control system indicates that adolescents may benefit from continued guidance in medical decision-making.[41]

Despite such arguments against allowing adolescents to make their own medical decisions in general, in matters related to sexual and reproductive health, minor patients are afforded the opportunity to assume decisional capacity and make autonomous decisions. Certainly, some adolescents may incorrectly calculate risks posed by divulging information to their parents, inaccurately assuming their parents to be oppositional when they would have been supportive. Others may overestimate the short-term harms of disclosure, fearing their parents' anger or disappointment and underestimating potential long-term benefits of disclosure, such as opening new lines of communication. While these laws may fail to address these subtleties, they act to protect those minors who correctly calculate significant harms of disclosure and would defer care were disclosure be mandated.

Conversations around sexual and reproductive healthcare can create space for providers to explore the degrees to which their adolescent patients may or may not be mature enough to make sound medical decisions for themselves. Such conversations help to illustrate that not all adolescents are alike—some 15-year-old patients will have the intellectual and emotional maturity to thoughtfully and easily weigh several medical options and determine the best course for them, and other 15-year-olds will require much more guidance and hand-holding by providers and/or family members during medical decision-making. This speaks to the idea that adolescents have emerging or graduated decision-making capacity: adolescents are actively developing their independent moral selves.[42,43] Adolescents mature physically at different rates, and they also mature cognitively, morally, and ethically at different rates.[41-43] Furthermore, although laws allow adolescents to consent for certain reproductive health services, a provider who deems that a minor lacks capacity to make certain decisions may determine it to be in the patient's best interest to include an adult family member in such decision-making.

Assessing decision-making capacity among adolescent patients who have varying degrees of capacity can be challenging for healthcare providers.[44] While some assessment tools to assess decision-making capacity exist, including the MacArthur Competence Assessment Tool for Treatment (Mac-CAT-T), such tools have not been fully validated with adolescents.[44] However, difficulties in assessing capacity are not limited to adolescent patients, as adult patients can also have varying degrees of decision-making capacity due to medical conditions or other circumstances. A sliding-scale framework helps to address questions of decision-making capacity in both adolescents and adults.[38,42,43] According to this framework, the decisional capacity threshold for making a high-risk, low-reward decision, such as participating in a potentially risky clinical trial, may be higher than the threshold required for making a low-risk, high-reward decision, such as testing for sexually transmitted infections.

Of course, counseling around all medical decisions should be thorough and assess patients' comprehension of key considerations. The sliding-scale framework, however, posits that the degree to which a healthcare provider can presume a patient's decision-making capacity or should scrutinize a patient's capacity depends on the risk–benefit ratio of the medical decision.[42,43] The sliding-scale framework is consistent with the mature minor doctrine (discussed earlier) that recognizes providers' ability to provide mainstream care that entails minimal risk to minors who demonstrate appropriate decision-making capacity.[1,8] The provision of reproductive health services, such as sexually transmitted disease testing, intrauterine devices and contraceptive implants, prenatal care, and pregnancy termination, meet the criteria of low-risk, high-reward care that falls within mainstream care and abides by both the sliding-scale framework and the mature minor doctrine.

Return to Clinical Case Addressing Consent and Confidentiality in Adolescent Reproductive Healthcare

1. How can providers navigate confidentiality obligations with minor patients?

Dr. Smith's first error was her failure to follow professional guidelines on upfront communication with Nina and her grandmother about consent and confidentiality. An essential first step in providing reproductive healthcare to adolescent patients is to have a candid conversation about confidentiality at the first adolescent visit. Preferably, this conversation should take place with an adult family member present to ensure transparency and foster trust between the healthcare provider, adolescent patient, and adult family member. Providers should explain in which situations the adolescent has a right to consent, and restrictions to the confidential nature of the patient–provider relationship. The legal restrictions vary by state but usually pertain to situations suggesting imminent danger to the adolescent themselves or to others at the hands of the adolescent, suspicion of evidence of abuse, and the diagnosis of certain communicable diseases.[34] Additionally, as was the case with Nina and her grandmother, providers should create the expectation that adult family members will be asked to step out of the clinical room at some point in the visit in order to create space for providers to speak privately with patients and allow them to ask questions that may be uncomfortable to ask in the presence of a family member. Furthermore, this conversation is an opportunity to educate parents about the importance of allowing their adolescent child to develop decision-making skills as they advance to adulthood. In situations in which the adolescent patient does not have a legal right to consent, but the clinician feels it is developmentally appropriate for this patient to do so, the clinician can ask the parent to allow it. At times parents will reject the premise that their adolescent child should have the right to privacy and consent and threaten to find a different provider. Reiterating that this is a legal standard and not a personal policy can be helpful in such circumstances to communicate that these rules apply to all adolescents and are not a value judgment about the parent and/or their child.

While Nina is 16 years old, these considerations may be different for a patient presenting under similar circumstances at the age of 11 years. Both according to state laws and based on socioemotional and cognitive development, allowing a young minor to make decisions independently from a parent may be inappropriate. Though such scenarios are thankfully rare, they do exist. A full discussion of how to address these cases is outside of the scope of this text. However, we strongly recommend enlisting additional experts, such as social workers and child life experts, to help address the needs of such a young minor and to assess for safety and home resources.

2. How can providers navigate conflicts with a minor patient's parent?

Nina's statutory right to consent to care (assuming she lives in a state in which she has one) does not mean Dr. Smith should automatically dismiss her mother from the equation. While adolescents have rights to confidentiality in accessing some sexual and reproductive healthcare, providers should seek to foster communication between their adolescent patients and adult family members in healthcare decisions when that is in the patient's best interest. For example, should a provider deem an adolescent not capable of making certain decisions due to the inability to comprehend risks, benefits, or alternatives to treatment options, they may determine it to be in the adolescent's best interest to include family in decision-making. Professional organizations emphasize the importance of promoting communication between adolescents and their parents or other caregivers when possible.[32–36] Adolescent providers frequently counsel adolescents about the advantages of including their parents/caregivers in medical decision-making. However, they also generally support an adolescent's desire to exclude their parents from decision-making when the patient concludes it would be detrimental to their health or well-being. Research shows that approximately half of adolescents seeking reproductive health services report that their parents were aware they were seeking this care.[29,44–48] For example, the majority of minors seeking abortion services do so with their parents' knowledge. Henshaw et al. found that 61% of young women discussed the decision to have an abortion with at least one of their parents.[49] Many adolescents who do not voluntarily discuss reproductive health decisions with their parents report compelling reasons for not doing so. Henshaw and colleagues found that 22% of teens who did not tell a parent about their abortion decision feared that they would be kicked out of the house if they told their parents about their decision. Approximately 8% of teens in this study feared that telling their parents would result in physical abuse, based on prior experiences with abuse at the hands of their parents. Providers should recognize that adolescent girls do involve their parents or caregivers in reproductive decision-making when they feel they can do so. Strategies for fostering parent–patient communication may include discussing with adolescent patients their perceptions of the pros and cons of communicating with parents, helping the adolescent see any potential advantages of increased parental communication, and offering to facilitate communication if the adolescent thinks this would be helpful. At the same time, when an adolescent patient expresses concerns about how their adult family member would respond or indicates that they would avoid care out of concern that her adult family member would be told of any results or findings, providers should prioritize the immediate healthcare needs of their patient.

3. What must providers consider in order to protect a minor patient's confidentiality?

Healthcare providers can control what they personally disclose to an adolescent's adult family member, but they may not have control over other parties' communications, such as detailed billing statements, printed after-visit summaries, and/or Explanation of Benefit notices sent by healthcare organizations and insurers to the parents/guarantors. These limitations should be disclosed to the patient as well. For example, when discussing potential lab testing and prescriptions, Dr. Smith should have explained to Nina that billing and diagnosis codes may show up on these documents. Parents and caregivers may also have proxy access to adolescent medical records on electronic medical records (EMR). Therefore, adolescents like Nina should be informed that some information, such as medications taken or prescribed and labs performed (i.e., test for sexually transmitted infections or pregnancy testing) could appear on the EMR and may be viewed by parents and guardians.[50] Additional suggestions for protecting a patient's confidentiality are outlined later.

4. How can providers improve systems and structures to support confidential care for a minor patient?

To begin with, healthcare providers serving adolescents should be knowledgeable about the laws and regulations governing their practice. Considering the important role that confidentiality plays for minors seeking healthcare, providers have an ethical duty to know how office and insurance procedures play out in practice and to advocate for changing those procedures to be more protective of adolescent confidentiality when possible. Providers should work to develop policies and protocols for staff, patients, and parents that include information regarding the scope and limitations of confidentiality, guidelines for payment of services, medical chart access, appointment scheduling, and information disclosure.[15]

Setting Expectations

It is crucial for providers to discuss at the first reproductive health visit an adolescent's right to confidentiality about certain topics and potential limitations to confidentiality. These issues should also be revisited in subsequent visits, especially when a provider may be recommending testing or prescribing medications related to sexual and reproductive health. Whether or not a test or treatment can be kept confidential is "material" to an adolescent patient's consent for that test or treatment, and, if that information is not provided, the patient cannot give informed consent or informed refusal to that test or treatment. For example, discussing with Nina that charges for pregnancy or sexually transmitted infection testing may come up on her mother's insurance bill may inform whether or not she would proceed with testing at your office.

Confidentiality in EMR

Given the potential challenges to ensuring confidentiality, it is important for providers who treat adolescents to call their EMR vendors to ensure that portals are properly configured to meet state standards regarding adolescent confidentiality. If the EMR system does not allow for accommodations to maintain adolescent confidentiality, the healthcare provider or staff should inform the patient that parents will have access to the records, and the patient should be given the option for referral to a healthcare provider who is required to provide confidential care, such as one who participates in the Title X family planning program. When test results come in, providers should strive to discuss such results directly with the patient.

Prescriptions

When Dr. Smith prescribed Nina azithromycin to treat her chlamydia, she should have asked Nina for her preferred pharmacy. Providers could also ask the pharmacy to call patients when a prescription is ready, provide patients with a written prescription that they can fill themselves, or advise patients to seek care at a Title X Family Planning clinic that is able to ensure confidentiality.

Billing and Insurance

Even though many adolescents have insurance coverage, those seeking confidential care may not want to use their insurance to pay for services if documentation of the services (e.g., an explanation of benefits) will be sent to the policy holder, who is likely a parent or guardian. Nina was covered through her mother's insurance, but under the HIPAA Privacy Rule a minor using insurance as an "individual" may request that providers and healthcare plans communicate with him or her in a confidential manner (e.g., email or personal cell phone). They can also request that the information disclosed for treatment, payment, or other services be limited. Nina should have been informed that she was entitled to ask for this. However, there may be administrative hurdles to implementing such a plan unless there are effective protocols in place for both providers' offices and third-party payers.[15] Providers can work with their clinic to establish practices to ensure sensitive information is sent using a patient's preferred contact information and even offer assistance for a young person interested in asking their insurance plan to communicate directly with them.

Health Policy

Finally, providers can play an important role in advocating for state laws to broaden and clarify confidentiality protections for minors seeking sexual and reproductive healthcare. Currently, 13 states have provisions that serve to protect the confidentiality of individuals insured as dependents. Five states allow individuals insured as dependents to request confidential communications from their insurance provider via a written request; two states allow insurers to mail explanations of benefits (EOBs) directly to the patient or withhold the EOB if no balance is due.[51] Providers can contribute to discussions about how these laws affect their practice and how they could be improved.

In conclusion, providing confidential reproductive healthcare to minor patients can seem daunting, particularly in the age of EMRs and other technology platforms meant to ease patient communication and patient record-keeping. However, taking the time to establish protocols, review internal clinic processes, and hold regular conversations with patients and their caregivers can help to establish trust with a young patient that will ultimately support their health and well-being.

References

1. English A. Sexual and reproductive health care for adolescents: Legal rights and policy challenges. *Adolesc Med.* 2007;18(3):571–81.
2. Spear SJ, English A. Protecting confidentiality to safeguard adolescents' health: Finding common ground. *Contraception.* 2007;76(2):73–6.
3. Ford CA, Millstein SG, Halpern-Felsher BL, et al. Influence of physician confidentiality assurances on adolescents' willingness to disclose information and seek future healthcare. A randomized controlled trial. *JAMA.* 1997;278:1029–34.
4. English A, Bass L, Dame Boyle A, Eshragh F. *State Minor Consent Laws: A Summary.* 3rd ed. Chapel Hill, NC: Center for Adolescent Health & the Law; 2010.
5. Guttmacher Institute. State laws and policies: An overview of minors' consent laws. 2019 Jan 25. https://www.guttmacher.org/state-policy/explore/overview-minors-consent-law
6. *Carey v. Population Services International,* 431 US 678 (1977).
7. *Bellotti v. Baird,* 443 US 622 (1979).
8. Berlan E, Bravender T. Confidentiality, consent, and caring for the adolescent patient. *Curr Opin Pediatr.* 2009;21(4):450–6.
9. English A, Ford CA. The HIPAA privacy rule and adolescents: Legal questions and clinical challenges. *Perspect Sexual Reprod Health.* 2004;Sect. 80–6.
10. Rosenbaum S, Abramson S, MacTaggart P. Health information law in the context of minors. *Pediatrics.* 2009 Jan;123(Supplement 2):S116–S21.
11. Guttmacher Institute, An Overview of Consent to Reproductive Health Services by Young People. April 1, 2021. https://www.guttmacher.org/state-policy/explore/overview-minors-consent-law
12. 45 CFR 160 and 164.
13. English A, Mulligan A, Coleman C. Protecting patients' privacy in health insurance billing & claims: A perspective from six states. National Family Planning & Reproductive Health Association. 2017. https://www.confidentialandcovered.com/file/1-research/1.1-research--findings/State-Profiles-Overview_CC.pdf
14. Ford C, English A, Sigman G. Confidential health care for adolescents: Position paper of the Society for Adolescent Medicine. *J Adolesc Health.* 2004;35(2):160–7.
15. Protecting adolescents: Ensuring access to care and reporting sexual activity and abuse: Position paper of the American Academy of Family Physicians, the American Academy of Pediatrics, the American College of Obstetricians and Gynecologists, and the Society for Adolescent Medicine. *J Adolesc Health.* 2004;35(5):420–3.
16. Center for Adolescent Health & the Law; Healthy Teen Network. Confidential contraceptive services for adolescents: What health care providers need to know about the law. 2006. http://www.cahl.org/PDFs/HelpingTeensStayHealthy&Save_Full%20Report.pdf
17. 42 USC. § 1396d(a)(4)(C).
18. 42 USC. § 1396a(a)(7).
19. 42 USC. § 300 et seq. 42 CFR Part 59. Program guidelines for project grants for family planning services. United States Department of Health and Human Services, Office of Public Health and Science, Office of Population Affairs, Office of Family Planning. 2001. http://www.hhs.gov/opa/pdfs/2001-ofp-guidelines.pdf

20. E.g., *T.H. v. Jones*, 425 F. Supp. 873 (D. Utah 1975), aff'd, 425 US 986 (1976) (finding violation of Supremacy Clause and Fourteenth Amendment); County of St. Charles, *Missouri v. Missouri Family Health Council*, 107 F. 3d 682, 684-85 (8th Cir. 1997); *Planned Parenthood Ass'n v. Dandoy*, 810 F.2d 984, 986-88 (10th Cir. 1987); *Jane Does 1 through 4 v. Utah Dep't of Health*, 776 F.2d 253, 255 (10th Cir. 1985); *New York v. Heckler*, 719 F.2d 1191, 1196 (2d Cir. 1983); *Planned Parenthood Fed'n v. Heckler*, 712 F.2d 650, 656-63 (D.C. Cir. 1983).

21. Boonstra H. Teen pregnancy: Trends and lessons learned. Guttmacher Report on Public Policy. 2002 Feb. http://www.guttmacher.org/pubs/tgr/05/1/gr050107.pdf

22. Torres A, Forrest JD. Family planning clinic services in the United States, 1981. *Fam Plann Perspect*. 1983 Nov–Dec;15(6):272–8.

23. Ventura SJ, Bachrach CA. Nonmarital childbearing in the United States, 1940–1999. *Natl Vital Stat Rep*. 2000;48(16):1–40. http://www.cdc.gov/nchs/data/nvsr48/nvs48_16.pdf

24. Moon M. Adolescents' right to consent to reproductive medical care: Balancing respect for families with public health goals. *AMA J Ethics*. 2012 Oct;14(10):805–8.

25. Abma JC, Martinez GM. *Sexual Activity and Contraceptive Use Among Teenagers in the United States, 2011–2015*. National Health Statistics Reports; no. 104. Hyattsville, MD: National Center for Health Statistics; 2017.

26. Centers for Disease Control and Prevention (CDC). Sexually transmitted disease surveillance 2014. US Department of Health and Human Services. 2015. https://www.cdc.gov/std/stats14/surv-2014-print.pdf

27. Kost K, Maddow-Zimet I, Arpaia A. Pregnancies, birth and abortions among adolescents and young women in the United States, 2013: National and state trends by age, race and ethnicity. https://www.guttmacher.org/report/us-adolescent-pregnancy-trends-2013

28. Boonstra HD. What is behind the declines in teen pregnancy rates? Summer 2014. https://www.guttmacher.org/gpr/2014/09/what-behind-declines-teen-pregnancy-rates

29. Reddy DM, Fleming R, Swain C. Effect of mandatory parental notification on adolescents girls' use of sexual health care services. *JAMA*. 2002 Aug;288(6):710–14.

30. Ford C, Bearman P, Moody J. Foregone health care among adolescents. *JAMA*. 1999,282:2227–34.

31. Fuentes L, Ingerick M, Jones R, Lindberg L. Adolescents' and young adults' reports of barriers to confidential health care and receipt of contraceptive services. *J Adolesc Health*. 2018;62:36–43.

32. American Medical Association (AMA). Ethics–5.055 Confidential care for minors. http://journalofethics.ama-assn.org/2014/11/coet1-1411.html

33. ACOG Committee on Adolescent Health Care. Confidentiality in Adolescent Health Care, Opinion Number 803. April 2020. https://www.acog.org/clinical/clinical-guidance/committee-opinion/articles/2020/04/confidentiality-in-adolescent-health-care

34. American Academy of Family Physicians (AAFP). Adolescent health care, confidentiality. http://www.aafp.org/about/policies/all/adolescent-confidentiality.html

35. American Academy of Pediatrics (AAP). Adolescent sexual health: Confidential services and private time. https://www.aap.org/en-us/advocacy-and-policy/aap-health-initiatives/adolescent-sexual-health/Pages/Confidential-Services-and-Private-Time.aspx

36. Ford C, English A, Sigman G. Confidential health care for adolescents: Position paper of the Society for Adolescent Medicine. *J Adolesc Health*. 2004;35:160–7.
37. Beauchamp TL, Childress JF. *Principles of Biomedical Ethics*. 7th ed. New York: Oxford University Press; 2012.
38. Johnson AR, Siegler M, Winslade WJ. *Clinical Ethics: A Practical Approach to Ethical Decisions in Clinical Medicine*. 8th ed. New York: McGraw-Hill Education; 2015.
39. Mercurio MR. Pediatric obstetrical ethics: Medical decision-making by, with, and for pregnant early adolescents. *Semin Perinatol*. 2016;40:237–46.
40. Ross LF. Against the tide: Arguments against respecting a minor's refusal of efficacious life-saving treatment. *Camb Q Healthc Ethics*. 2009;18:315–22.
41. Grootens-Wiegers P, Hein IM, Van den Broek JM, de Vries MC. Medical decision-making in children and adolescents: Developmental and neuroscientific aspects. *BMC Pediatrics*. 2017;17:120.
42. Levine C, Blustein J, Dubler NN. Introduction: The adolescent alone: "You got nobody in your corner." In Blustein J, Levine C, Dubler NN, eds., *The Adolescent Alone: Decision Making in Health Care in the United States*. Cambridge: Cambridge University Press; 1999:1–20.
43. Blustein J, Moreno JD. Valid consent to treatment and the unsupervised adolescent. In Blustein J, Levine C, Dubler NN, eds., *The Adolescent Alone: Decision Making in Health Care in the United States*. Cambridge: Cambridge University Press; 1999:100–110.
44. Hein IM, Troost PW, Broersma A, de Vries MC, Daams JG, Lindauer RJ. Why is it hard to make progress in assessing children's decision-making competence? *BMC Med Ethics*. 2015;16:1.
45. Jones RK, Purcell A, Singh S, et al. Adolescents' reports of parental knowledge of adolescents' use of sexual health services and their reactions to parental notification for prescription contraception. *JAMA*. 2002;2932(3):710–14.
46. Nathanson CA, Becker MH. Family and peer influence on obtaining a method of contraception. *J Marriage Fam*. 1986;48:513–25.
47. Torres A. Does your mother know? *Fam Plann Perspect*. 1978;10:280–2.
48. Hasselbacher LA, Dekleva A, Tristan S, Gilliam M. Factors influencing parental involvement among minors seeking and abortion: A qualitative study. *AJPH*. 2014;104:2207–11.
49. Henshaw SK, Kost K. Parental involvement in minors' abortion decisions. *Fam Plann Perspect*. 1992;24:196–207, 213.
50. Stablein T, Loud KJ, DiCapua C, Anthony DL. The catch to confidentiality: The use of electronic health records in adolescent health care. *J Adolesc Health*. 2018;62:577–82.
51. Guttmacher Institute. State laws and policies: Protecting confidentiality for individuals insured as dependents. 2019 Jan 25. https://www.guttmacher.org/state-policy/explore/protecting-confidentiality-individuals-insured-dependents

4

Contraception and Abortion in the United States

A Brief Legal History

David A. Strauss JD

The Common Law and the Nineteenth Century

The law governing abortion in the United States—like much of US law—has its origins in the common law of England. The common law was judge-made law, derived from precedents and social practices. It was carried into the Colonies, and then, after the American Revolution, it continued as the law of the new states. According to the common law, the legally significant point in the development of the fetus was "quickening"—the first time a pregnant woman could perceive the fetus in her body. William Blackstone's *Commentaries on the Laws of England*, the mid-eighteenth-century treatise that was the authoritative account of the common law in the Colonies and new states, said that life "begins in contemplation of law as soon as an infant is able to stir in the mother's womb."[1] The quickening doctrine had ancient roots; it seems to have been established in England as early as the thirteenth century.[2]

According to the common law, an abortion performed before quickening was not unlawful.[3] After quickening, it was a crime to induce an abortion, but "the crime was qualitatively different from the destruction of human being . . . and [was] punished less harshly."[4] Because records are incomplete, it is difficult to know how often people were prosecuted, or punished, for this crime. But, in any event, "American women in 1800 were legally free to attempt to terminate a condition that might turn out to have been a pregnancy until the existence of that pregnancy was incontrovertibly confirmed by the perception of fetal movement."[5] English law took a more restrictive turn in 1803, when Parliament made it a crime to have an abortion before quickening, but US law did not follow. In 1812, the highest court in Massachusetts ruled, consistent with common law principles, that an alleged abortionist could not be prosecuted because there was no allegation " 'that the woman was quick with child at the time.'"[6] That precedent was followed in most states through the first half of the nineteenth century, and in some places for years after that.[7]

Beginning in the 1820s, some state legislatures began to enact laws on abortion that modified the common law principles. In 1821, Connecticut enacted a statute making it a crime to cause a woman to take " 'any deadly poison, or other noxious and destructive substance, with an intention . . . thereby to . . . cause or procure the miscarriage of any woman, then being quick with child.' "[8] A few other states enacted similar laws in the next few years.[9] The Connecticut law made no effort to outlaw abortion pre-quickening; in that respect, it maintained the nonrestrictive features of the common law. The Connecticut statute, and others like it, did not make it a crime to have an abortion—only to administer an abortifacient or to cause it to be taken. So the pregnant woman herself would not commit a crime, under this statute, by having an abortion. In fact, the law seems to have been concerned primarily with the harm that an abortifacient might cause to the woman and only secondarily with abortion.[10]

By 1841, 10 states (of the 26 then in the Union) had laws dealing with abortion; those laws generally conformed to the pattern set by the Connecticut law. Half of them maintained the line that the common law set at quickening, and they reflected the "judgment . . . that women who sought abortions even post-quickening were not themselves criminals, but 'victims of their own moral weakness who needed state protection.' "[11] Five states' laws did outlaw pre-quickening abortions, but, to the extent they did so, they were probably unenforceable, perhaps intentionally so: those laws required a showing that the woman was pregnant or that there was intent to cause a miscarriage. Before quickening, it was, in practice, likely to be impossible to show either of those things with the certainty needed for a criminal conviction.[12]

States began to adopt more restrictive laws in the 1840s, after the Second Great Awakening, the Protestant religious revival of the first decades of the nineteenth century. In 1845, New York enacted a law that was directed squarely at women, that was not limited to post-quickening abortions, and that covered all means of obtaining abortions. It provided that "[e]very woman who shall solicit" any abortifacient or who "shall submit to any operation" with the intent "to procure a miscarriage" would be guilty of a crime.

But not a serious crime: even that New York law, which was notably more restrictive than the common law, said that a woman who obtained an abortion was guilty of only a misdemeanor.[13] And although other states followed New York in modifying the common law in the 1840s and 1850s, few of those state statutes were as were as restrictive as New York's. Thirteen of the 33 states had no statutes prohibiting abortion on their books; they adhered to the common law regime. Most other states maintained the immunity for pre-quickening abortions.[14]

The real change began in the 1860s. Between 1860 and 1880, the United States saw "the most important burst of anti-abortion legislation in the nation's history."[15] The leading history of nineteenth-century abortion laws describes it this way:

> At least 40 anti-abortion statutes of various kinds were placed upon state and territorial lawbooks [between 1860 and 1880]; over 30 in the years from 1866 through 1877 alone. Some 13 jurisdictions formally outlawed abortion for the first time, and at least 21 states revised their already existing statutes on the subject. More significantly, most of the legislation passed between 1860 and 1880 explicitly accepted the [premise] . . . that the interruption of gestation at any point in a pregnancy should be a crime.[16]

This change in US law was a lasting one. The laws enacted during this period set the tone for the next hundred years,[17] until the wave of abortion reform in the 1960s and 1970s. "Some of the laws passed during this period remained literally unchanged through the 1960s; others were altered only in legal phraseology, not in basic philosophy."[18]

Many factors undoubtedly contributed to this dramatic change, but one stands out: beginning in the 1850s, the fledgling American Medical Association (AMA) "launched an aggressive campaign to rid the nation of abortion."[19] The AMA established a "Committee on Criminal Abortion"; the Committee's recommendations were ultimately accepted by the AMA as a whole. Horatio Storer, a Boston gynecologist who chaired the committee, "insisted that women must remain within their 'God-given sphere.'"[20] The Committee asserted that abortion should be forbidden at every point in a pregnancy "'except as necessary for preserving the life of the mother'" and that the determination whether the mother's life was endangered could be made only by a doctor.[21] The Committee's arguments anticipated justifications for limiting abortion that are made in litigation to this day: that "'the foetus in utero is alive from the very moment of conception'" and that abortion presents a danger to women's physical and mental well-being.[22] The AMA, together with medical journals and state and local medical societies, campaigned throughout the nation for restrictions on abortion.[23]

As far as the law was concerned, the campaign could not have been more successful. By the end of the nineteenth century, every state had outlawed abortion unless a doctor stated that an abortion was needed to save the woman's life.[24] The line that the common law had drawn at quickening disappeared; the new wave of laws applied both pre- and post-quickening. Women who sought abortions could be prosecuted. At the same time, governments tried to prevent information about abortions from reaching people who might seek it.[25] And the law remained essentially in this state until the middle of the twentieth century.

But, in another respect, the campaign against abortion, and the restrictive laws it precipitated, were not so successful. Reliable statistics on illegal abortions are hard to come by, for obvious reasons. But, according to plausible estimates, by the middle of the twentieth century there were about 1 million abortions annually in the United States.[26] Although nearly all the abortions performed in the United States at that time were illegal, women with resources could get abortions by traveling to countries that allowed abortions or by connecting with a network of doctors who would, for a price, perform abortions clandestinely. Women without resources risked serious injuries. Those factors, and others, led to efforts to reform abortion laws beginning in the 1960s.[27] At first, reform efforts focused on state legislatures; later, they turned to the courts.

Legislative Reform in the Twentieth Century

The first important step toward liberalizing abortion laws was taken by the American Law Institute (ALI). The ALI is a group of lawyers, judges, and academics who are prominent in the profession; among other things, the ALI suggests ways to systematize the law and bring it up to date, and it drafts "model laws"—proposed statutes that state legislatures might use in revising the laws on their books. The Model Penal Code (MPC), a proposed revision of the criminal law, was one of the ALI's most prominent projects.

In 1962, as part of the MPC, the ALI proposed that abortion laws be liberalized by allowing what came to be called "therapeutic abortions." The MPC was written in terms of providing legal protection for doctors who performed abortions—it provided the circumstances in which "[a] physician is justified in terminating a pregnancy"—rather than in terms of establishing the rights of women, although the effect of protecting doctors was that women would be able to obtain abortions. The MPC provided that a physician who believed that there was "a substantial risk" that continuing the pregnancy "would gravely impair the physical or mental health of the mother" could terminate the pregnancy. In addition, an abortion would be justified if the doctor believed "that the child would be born with grave mental or physical defect, or that the pregnancy resulted from rape, incest, or other felonious intercourse."[28] Consistent with the MPC's focus on physicians' prerogatives, the model statute provided that "[no] abortion shall be performed" unless two physicians "certified in writing the circumstances" that justified the abortion.[29]

Between 1967 and 1970, 12 states liberalized their abortion laws by adopting statutes that followed, to varying degrees, the ALI recommendation.[30] They allowed therapeutic abortions but generally required that a physician, or sometimes a panel of physicians, certify that the criteria for therapeutic abortions were met. In 1970, four states—Alaska, Hawaii, Washington, and New York—went further: they repealed the existing laws forbidding abortions and allowed women to end a pregnancy for any reason, up to a certain gestational age.[31]

But at that point—in 1970—efforts to liberalize abortion law in state legislatures stalled. No reform measures were adopted between 1970 and 1972. New York's liberalizing law was nearly repealed: a repeal measure passed the legislature, but Governor Nelson Rockefeller vetoed it.[32] In 1972, in what some proponents of abortion liberalization regarded as "a terrible blow," a referendum proposal that would have liberalized Michigan's abortion laws was defeated.[33] In two-thirds of the states, abortions were still illegal unless carrying the pregnancy to term would endanger the woman's life. Reform advocates turned to litigation, rather than legislation, to try to accomplish their goals. Cases asserting that state laws banning abortion were unconstitutional were brought in court. In fact, by 1972, the case that would become *Roe v. Wade* was already before the Supreme Court.

The Constitutional Law of Abortion

The foundation of the constitutional law governing abortion was laid in a case, decided in 1965, that did not involve abortion and that, in retrospect—considering the controversy that continues to surround *Roe v. Wade*[34]—seems remarkably one-sided. The case, *Griswold v. Connecticut*,[35] was a challenge to the constitutionality of a Connecticut law that prohibited the use of contraceptives for the purpose of birth control by any person, married or single. Unlike other laws prohibiting the sale or distribution of contraceptives, the Connecticut statute banned the use of contraceptives—a private and intimate act. It applied to married couples.[36] And because it forbade the use of contraceptives only for birth control and not to prevent disease, it could be easily evaded by individuals (men who used condoms and women who could convince their partners to do so), although it was enforced against birth control clinics. Even one of the Supreme Court Justices who believed that the statute was constitutional—Justice Potter Stewart—suggested that it was "asinine."[37]

A majority of the Court held that the statute was unconstitutional. That decision was not controversial outside the Court.[38] But for reasons peculiar to the history of American constitutional law, it was in some ways a groundbreaking decision. When *Roe v. Wade* came before the Court a few years later, some of the Justices tended to see *Roe* as simply the next step after *Griswold*, not as what *Roe* would prove to be—a vastly more controversial and divisive decision.

Griswold seemed to be a turning point because the Court relied on a constitutional right—a right to "privacy," as the Court characterized it—that had no clear basis in the text of the Constitution, unlike, for example, rights to freedom of speech or freedom of religion, which are mentioned in terms in the First Amendment. In the first three decades of the twentieth century, the Supreme Court had invoked rights to economic freedom, which also lacked a clear basis in the text, as a way of invalidating social welfare and regulatory legislation—minimum wage laws, maximum hour laws, occupational licensing laws, and the like. Many people, in and out of government, thought those laws were critical means of adapting to the emerging industrial economy of the United States, and increasingly the Court came under attack. When new Supreme Court justices repudiated those early-twentieth-century decisions during President Franklin Roosevelt's New Deal, one of their rallying cries was that the Supreme Court should never again "invent" rights that were not clearly stated in the text of the Constitution. But then *Griswold*, with its right to privacy, seemed to do just that, only with a different right—privacy, instead of economic liberty. The dissenting justices in *Griswold* thought that was a betrayal of the lesson learned in Roosevelt's time. But a majority of the Court was comfortable recognizing a right to privacy that had no clear basis in the text of the Constitution.

When *Roe* came before the Court, it was, for that reason, natural to think that *Griswold* had taken the big step—establishing a right to privacy—and *Roe* was just a follow-on, a matter of implementing that right. The Court's preoccupation with "invented" rights obscured from its view the truly divisive issues in the abortion debate: the equality of women, on one side, and the status of fetal life, on the other.[39] But even apart from the background in constitutional law, the justices had reason to think that *Roe* would not be particularly controversial. Public opinion polls showed widespread agreement with the statement "The decision to have an abortion should be made solely by a woman and her physician." Overall, 64% of respondents agreed and 31% disagreed; there was majority support among Catholics, Republicans, and Democrats (more support among Republicans than among Democrats, in fact).[40]

Roe, which was decided in January 1973, revolutionized the law of abortion in the United States. The Court ruled that the Constitution guaranteed the right to have an abortion, free from restrictions imposed by state law, in the first trimester of a pregnancy. During the second trimester, abortion could be regulated, but only in order to protect the health of the woman. Once the fetus was viable, a state could, if it wished, forbid abortion, unless an abortion was necessary to preserve the life or health of the mother.[41] Within the Court, the decision was not especially hard-fought: a 7–2 majority voted to strike down the Texas abortion law at issue in the case. And, as the public opinion polls suggested, *Roe* was not instantly controversial outside the Court.[42]

Within a few years, though, opposition to the decision began to build. In 1977, the Court upheld a Connecticut law that said Medicaid funds could not be used for abortions that were not "medically necessary."[43] Three years later, the Court went further and upheld the federal statute known as the Hyde Amendment, which prohibited the use of federal funds for abortions even when they were needed to protect the health of the mother.[44] By this time, *Roe*'s critics had begun a concerted campaign to overturn the decision, focusing particularly on appointments to the Supreme Court. By 1991, only one member of the seven-justice majority that voted in favor of the result in *Roe*—Justice Harry Blackmun, the author of the opinion of the Court in *Roe*—remained on the Supreme Court; several of his colleagues had been replaced by presidents who had expressed their opposition to abortion rights. Some of those justices explicitly called for the Court to overrule *Roe*.

In 1989, the Court came close to doing so. It upheld a Missouri law that imposed a variety of limits on the right to an abortion—for example, a ban on abortions in public hospitals—and four justices, one short of a majority, strongly hinted that *Roe* should be overruled. Justice Blackmun wrote an impassioned opinion warning that the right to an abortion might not survive much longer.[45] But in 1992, the Court, somewhat surprisingly, declined to abolish the right to an abortion and reaffirmed important aspects of *Roe*.

The 1992 decision, *Planned Parenthood of Southeast Pennsylvania v. Casey*,[46] established the framework for evaluating laws regulating abortion that has survived to this day—although possibly only in name. *Casey* rejected the trimester approach of *Roe* but continued to draw a line at viability. After viability, a state could forbid abortion as long as it allowed an exception for the life and health of the woman. Before viability, a state could not ban abortion, but it could regulate abortion. A regulation would be constitutional if it did not impose an "undue burden" on the right to an abortion.[47] That term—"undue burden"—continues to be the main criterion for determining whether laws limiting the right to an abortion are constitutional.

But "undue burden" is a vague term, and the Court's definition of "undue burden" did not help very much. An undue burden, the Court said, exists when a "state regulation has the purpose or effect of placing a substantial obstacle in the path of a woman seeking an abortion of a nonviable fetus."[48] "Substantial obstacle" is not much more precise than "undue burden." And although the reference to "purpose" suggested that it would matter whether a law was passed because the legislature was hostile to abortion, the Court has not followed up on that suggestion; it has not looked into the motivations behind laws that restricted abortion.

The vagueness of the "undue burden" test left the door open for states that are hostile to the right to abortion to enact laws that make it increasingly difficult for women to exercise that right, and, increasingly, states have done so.[49] In general, state regulations of abortions have taken two forms.[50] Some claim to be justified by the state's interest in recognizing the value of fetal life, an interest that the Supreme Court, in *Casey*, explicitly said a state may assert by favoring childbirth over abortion.[51] Laws imposing waiting periods on women seeking abortions or counseling requirements on abortion providers are examples. The other category of laws purports to be concerned with women's well-being. These regulations—which proponents of abortion rights call TRAP laws, for "targeted regulation of abortion providers"— typically require that facilities offering abortions conform to relatively onerous requirements or that abortion providers have certain qualifications. Recently, opponents of abortion seem increasingly to favor the latter kind of laws—so-called TRAP laws—as a means of limiting access to abortion.[52]

In 2016, the Supreme Court, *Whole Woman's Health v. Hellerstedt*,[53] struck down two such laws that had been enacted by Texas. One law required abortion facilities to meet the standards that Texas sets for ambulatory surgical centers; another required physicians who provided abortions to have admitting privileges at a nearby hospital. The Court looked closely at the specific facts about how the Texas laws operated—how many abortion clinics would have to close as a result of the laws, how far women would have to travel as a result, whether the admitting privileges requirement would be likely to improve health outcomes. The Court applied a kind of cost–benefit analysis. It determined that the benefits of the Texas requirements were minimal or nonexistent and were easily outweighed by the burden imposed on women seeking abortions.

But a lot has happened since *Whole Woman's Health*, and at this point the future of abortion rights in the United States is very uncertain. Since the Presidential election of 2016, the composition of both the Supreme Court and the lower federal courts has changed dramatically. Only four members of the majority in *Whole Woman's Health* remain on the Court, and the new appointees are expected to be strongly opposed to abortion rights. Many judges who have been openly opposed to abortion rights have been appointed to the lower courts as well.

June Medical Services v. Russo,[54] a 2020 Supreme Court decision, shows just how uncertain abortion rights have become. The case involved a Louisiana state law that imposed an admitting privileges requirement; the Louisiana law was nearly a carbon copy of the Texas law that *Whole Woman's Health* had declared unconstitutional. Ordinarily, a law that is inconsistent with a recent Supreme Court decision will be quickly struck down by the lower courts, which are obligated to follow Supreme Court decisions whether they agree with them or not. If a lower court does not do that, it can expect to be sharply rebuked by the Supreme Court, which usually does not hesitate to assert its authority.[55] But in *June Medical*, a lower court upheld the Louisiana law. The Supreme Court ultimately declared the Louisiana law unconstitutional, but it did not rebuke the lower court, and the decision may have left *Whole Woman's Health* in limbo. The vote in *June Medical* was 5–4; Chief Justice Roberts, who had dissented in *Whole Woman's Health*, cast the decisive vote, saying that he believed the Court should follow its precedent. But he asserted that under the "undue burden" approach, the Court should consider only the burden imposed by a regulation—not whether it provided any benefit.

The effect of *June Medical*, despite its bottom-line outcome, will be to encourage states that want to limit women's ability to obtain abortions to keep trying more and more severe restrictions. The Chief Justice's opinion, combined with the vagueness of the "undue burden" standard, gives lower court judges leeway to uphold laws that serve hardly any purpose except to make it harder to get an abortion. The Supreme Court's failure to rebuke the lower court invites lower court judges who are hostile to abortion rights to be increasingly aggressive in pushing the boundaries that the Supreme Court has established.[56] The most likely scenario, given the current composition of the Supreme Court, is that even if the formal "undue burden" standard remains in place, there will be an increasing erosion of the right to an abortion. In states that are determined to limit abortion rights, the result might not be any different in practice from what it would be if *Roe v. Wade* had never been decided.

Other possible scenarios are even less favorable to abortion rights. The long-running effort to overrule *Roe v. Wade*, and now *Casey*, might finally succeed. The effect would be that states would be free simply to make abortions unlawful, and abortion rights would be determined entirely by the law of particular states. One plausible speculation, though, is that as long as the courts continue to uphold increasingly restrictive state limits on abortion rights, there is no reason for justices opposed to abortion rights to overrule *Roe* and *Casey* formally, something that would be much more controversial politically than the continued erosion of those rights. In one extreme scenario—very unlikely, but not completely out of the question—the Court might decide that it is unconstitutional not to protect fetal life, so that the Constitution would require that abortion be prohibited throughout the United States. A movement in the other direction—making abortion rights more secure—would require the appointment of justices who viewed abortion rights more favorably than do the current members of the Court.

Conclusion

On the surface, the history of the law of abortion in the United States is a history of pendulum swings. The relatively liberal common law regime was followed by the highly restrictive laws imposed in the late nineteenth century. The legislative reforms of the 1960s undid some of those laws, although that reform movement stopped abruptly. The establishment of a constitutional right to abortion in *Roe v. Wade* liberalized abortion laws again, but the right that *Roe* recognized was limited in the years that followed. *Casey* rebuffed efforts to overrule *Roe*, but it allowed state restrictions that complied with the "undue burden" standard. *Whole Woman's Health* seemed to reinvigorate the right to an abortion, but *June Medical*, reflecting changes in the courts, foreshadows a sharp movement in the other direction.

One unfortunate constant, however, seems to be that a woman's ability to have an abortion will depend on arbitrary factors. Increasingly, given the propensity of some states to enact severe restrictions and the courts' willingness to allow them to do so, it depends on whether a woman lives in a place that has restrictive laws. Beyond that, social norms and practices that make abortion unavailable as a practical matter can be just as effective as legal restrictions in preventing access to an abortion. At the same time, some women will be well off enough, in financial or other resources, to overcome whatever restrictions exist, at least as long as abortion is legal in many places; but many others will not.

One of the most important missions of the law is to prevent the disagreements that inevitably arise among people, especially in a large and diverse nation, from undermining the fabric of society and individuals' well-being. Disagreements about abortion in the United States seem to be deeply rooted. It may be too much to expect the law to resolve them without leaving one side aggrieved. But it is hard to justify a resolution that imposes the costs of society's collective ambivalence on people who are already disadvantaged. To the extent that this is what our law has done, perhaps no one, whatever his or her views on abortion, should find it acceptable.

References

1. Blackstone W. 1 *Commentaries on the Laws of England*, asterisked note 129 (1765).
2. See Mohr JC. *Abortion in America: The Origins and Evolution of National Policy, 1800–1900*. New York: Oxford University Press;1976: 265 n. 1.

3. See Stone GR. *Sex and the Constitution: Sex, Religion, and Law from America's Origins to the Twenty-first Century*. New York: Liveright; 2017:) 184.

4. Mohr, *Abortion in America*, 3–4.

5. Ibid., 4.

6. Ibid., 5.

7. Ibid.

8. Ibid., 21, quoting The Public Statute Laws of the State of Connecticut, 1821 (Hartford, 1821), 152–3.

9. See Mohr, *Abortion in America*, 25–6.

10. See generally Ibid., 21–3.

11. Stone, *Sex and the Constitution*, 185; see also Mohr, *Abortion in America*, 137.

12. See Mohr, *Abortion in America*, 43.

13. See Means CC Jr. The law of New York concerning abortion and the status of the foetus, 1664–1968: A case of cessation of constitutionality. *NY Law Forum*. 1968;14:411, 454 n. 101. See generally Stone, *Sex and the Constitution*, 185–6.

14. See Mohr, *Abortion in America*, 145–6.

15. Ibid., 200.

16. Ibid.

17. Ibid., 200–1.

18. Ibid., 225.

19. Stone, *Sex and the Constitution*, 189. See generally Luker K. *Abortion and the Politics of Motherhood*. Berkeley: University of California Press; 1984: 15–36.

20. Stone, *Sex and the Constitution*, 189.

21. Ibid., 187.

22. Ibid., 188.

23. See Mohr, *Abortion in America*, 159.

24. See Reagan LJ. *When Abortion Was a Crime: Women, Medicine, and Law in the United States, 1867–1973*. Berkeley: University of California Press; 1997:) 5.

25. See Stone, *Sex and the Constitution*, 189.

26. See Calderone MS. Illegal abortion as a public health problem, *Am J Pub Health*. 1960;50: 948, 950, reprinted in Greenhouse L, Siegel RB, eds., *Before Roe v. Wade: Voices That Shaped the Abortion Debate Before the Supreme Court's Ruling*. New York: Kaplan; 2010: 23.

27. See Greenhouse and Siegel, *Before Roe v. Wade*, 3.

28. American Law Institute, Model Penal Code, Section 230.3 (1962), reprinted in Greenhouse and Siegel, *Before Roe v. Wade*, 25. The reference to children born with "grave physical or mental defect" was very likely a response to publicity surrounding children born with serious birth defects because their mothers had taken the drug thalidomide. See the accounts in, for example, Chessen Finkbine S. The lesser of two evils, reprinted in Greenhouse and Siegel, *Before Roe v. Wade*, 11–18; Garrow DJ, *Liberty & Sexuality: The Right to Privacy and the Making of Roe v. Wade*. New York: Macmillan; 1994: 285–9; Stone, *Sex and the Constitution*, 271–2.

29. Model Penal Code, Section 230.3(3), reprinted in Greenhouse and Siegel, *Before Roe v. Wade*, 25.

30. See Greenhouse and Siegel, *Before Roe v. Wade*, 24; Burns G. *The Moral Veto: Framing Contraception, Abortion, and Cultural Pluralism in the United States.* Cambridge: Cambridge University Press; 2005: 177 (table 5.1). A statute modeled on the ALI proposal was later declared unconstitutional in a case decided at the same time as *Roe v. Wade*. See *Doe v. Bolton*, 410 US 179 (1973).

31. Burns, *The Moral Veto*, 178 (table 5.3).

32. See Stone, *Sex and the Constitution*, 382; Greenhouse and Siegel, *Before Roe v. Wade*, 281 n. 69.

33. See Garrow, *Liberty and Sexuality*, 577.

34. 410 US 113 (1973).

35. 381 US 479 (1965).

36. In 1972, the Supreme Court, extending *Griswold*, declared unconstitutional a Massachusetts law that prohibited the distribution of contraceptives to unmarried people. See *Eisenstadt v. Baird*, 405 US 438 (1972).

37. 381 US at 527 (Stewart J, dissenting).

38. See, for example, Stone, *Sex and the Constitution*, 362–3.

39. For an elaboration of these points, see Strauss DA. Abortion, toleration, and moral uncertainty. *Supreme Court Rev.* 1992;1.

40. Gallup G. Abortion seen up to woman, doctor; reprinted in Greenhouse and Siegel, *Before Roe v. Wade*, 209.

41. 410 US at 163–5.

42. See Stone, *Sex and the Constitution*, 393–5.

43. *Maher v. Roe*, 432 US 464 (1977).

44. *Harris v. McRae*, 448 US 297 (1980).

45. *Webster v. Reproductive Health Services*, 492 US 490 (1989).

46. 505 US 833 (1992).

47. Ibid., 874 (opinion of Kennedy, O'Connor, Souter JJ).

48. Ibid., 877 (opinion of Kennedy, O'Connor, Souter JJ).

49. For a summary, see https://www.guttmacher.org/state-policy/explore/overview-abortion-laws

50. See Ziegler M. Substantial uncertainty: Whole Woman's Health v Hellerstedt and the future of abortion law. *Supreme Court Rev.* 2016;77.

51. 505 US at 875–6 (opinion of Kennedy, O'Connor, Souter JJ).

52. See Ziegler, Substantial uncertainty, 99–101, https://www.guttmacher.org/state-policy/explore/targeted-regulation-abortion-providers#

53. 136 S. Ct. 2292 (2016).

54. 140 S.Ct. 2013 (2020).

55. The advocates of abortion rights in *June Medical* reminded the Supreme Court of a recent example from another controversial area of constitutional law. Montana enacted a campaign finance law that seemed inconsistent with the Supreme Court's well-known (and widely criticized) decision in *Citizens United v. Federal Election Commission*, 558 US 310 (2010). The Montana Supreme Court upheld the law, reasoning that Montana's different circumstances justified a different result from what the Supreme Court had done in *Citizens United*. The Supreme Court summarily

overturned the Montana Supreme Court's decision in a brisk one-paragraph opinion. See *American Tradition Partnership, Inc. v. Bullock*, 567 US 516 (2012).

56. Within a few weeks after *June Medical* was decided, one lower court, following the Chief Justice's approach, had already ordered that restrictions on abortions must to be evaluated simply by considering the burdens they imposed, not by inquiring into whether they conferred any benefit, and that courts should be deferential to state legislatures in assessing those laws. See *Hopkins v. Jegley*, 2020 WL 4557687 (8th Cir. 2020).

SECTION II
ASSISTED REPRODUCTION ETHICS
Initiating Pregnancy

Overview

Assisted Reproduction Ethics

Katie Watson JD and Julie Chor MD, MPH

Many people move directly from this book's first topic to its third—from pregnancy prevention to conception and childbirth. Others who want to become pregnant find they need medical assistance to do so. Some people who receive these services are successful: in 2018, assisted reproductive technology (ART) treatments in the United States resulted in 73,831 live births and 81,478 infants, according to the Centers for Disease Control (CDC).[1] The fact that more than 60% of ART patients are of advanced maternal age (>35 years) illustrates just one of the ways this area of reproductive medicine is changing our social landscape.[2]

Radically different legal landscapes govern the medical interventions that help people prevent or end pregnancy, considered in Section I, and the medical interventions that help people create pregnancy, considered in this section. Contraception and abortion are the only types of healthcare that have been constitutionally protected, yet federal and state statutes have also made them the most restricted. This legal context is flipped in other areas of medicine: patients don't have a constitutional right to knee surgery, but legislatures don't restrict their ability to choose it or doctors' ability to provide it, beyond basic safety regulation. Legally, ART is treated more like knee surgery than abortion despite the fact that it also engages profound questions of human existence, and it creates and destroys a significant number of embryos. The US Supreme Court has not established an affirmative constitutional right to use medical interventions to create a pregnancy, but legislatures rarely restrict access to ART. (We say "rarely" because there are a few exceptions to the rule—for example, Michigan criminalizes compensated surrogacy contracts[3]—but in the vast majority of states access to ART is unfettered by the law.) What accounts for this legal difference between abortion and ART? Perhaps it is a product of an underlying cultural belief that women are meant to be mothers, and therefore medical practices that create babies and transform women into mothers will be permitted regardless of what is required to achieve this result.

However, not all motherhood is valued equally. In this section's first chapter (Chapter 5) physician-scholar Lisa H. Harris centers this justice issue, reviewing the history of in vitro fertilization (IVF)'s introduction in the 1980s and expansion to donor oocytes in the 1990s to understand how and why infertility has been constructed as an ailment of white professional women despite the fact black women are 1.5 to 2 times as likely to experience infertility as their white counterparts. Dr. Harris illuminates the ways race and class inequalities in the US are viscerally reproduced in and by our reproductive practices, and she argues that the central ethical issue in IVF care is the justice issue of how IVF reproduces stratified reproduction itself.

Ethics are at the forefront of everyday practice in ART because physicians have become gatekeepers who decide who may have babies and what those patients may and may not do to create babies. For example, in Chapter 6, law and ethics professor Valerie Gutmann Koch considers the ethical questions and legal liabilities for physicians and facilities that use preimplantation genetic testing (PGT) to screen and select for chromosomal abnormalities and genetic traits, and she explains the difference between informed consent, wrongful birth, and wrongful life claims.

Distinctive ethics issues are raised by ART that works with three people to make a baby: the 9% of ART cycles that intended to use eggs from a donor[4] and the almost 4% of all 2016 embryo transfers that went to a gestational surrogate.[5] In Chapter 7, ART lawyer Heather Ross analyzes the conflicts of interest and systematic bias that can occur when physicians treat both intended parents and the egg donor with whom they have partnered, and the ethical dilemmas that arise when a gestational surrogate and the intended parents with whom she has partnered disagree on medical choices affecting the fetus. In Chapter 8, ART psychologist Susan Klock considers the well-being of oocyte donors and the children they help create: Is paid "donation" voluntary? Is egg donation physically and psychologically safe? And how should clinicians help social parents navigate whether, when, and how to tell their child that an egg donor provided half of the child's genetic material?

A significant number of contemporary ART patients are fertile and not currently seeking pregnancy. Previously this category was comprised of egg donors, but in recent years a new type of patient has joined: those seeking to bank their own eggs or embryos for the future. Many of these cycles were for young women planning for the future, and some of them were cancer patients confronting fertility-threatening disease or treatment. In Chapter 9, scientists Teresa Woodruff, Jhenifer Rodrigues, and Bruno Ramahlo de Carvalho help clinicians understand the ethical issues unique to oncofertility, such as the assent process for pediatric cancer patients, and the posthumous use or destruction of gametes preserved by cancer patients who die before using them.

The section closes with physician-ethicist Veronique Fournier and legal scholar-ethicist Laurence Brunet's analysis of the ethical strengths and limitations of the French approach to ART, which returns us to the fact that every country's ART practice is a product of its cultural values (Chapter 10). For example, France's commitment to publicly funded healthcare is reflected in its choice to pay for all ART needed for "medical" reasons, and its rejection of commodification of human bodies is reflected in its choice to criminalize all surrogacy and any payment for gametes. However, France's total ban on ART for same-sex couples is now in tension with the respect for family autonomy reflected in its legalization of same-sex marriage.

Many practitioners are drawn to ART because of the enormous positive impact the field has on patient and family life. Some are also inspired by the field's complex ethical challenges, and every ob-gyn must be able to navigate them at some level. The chapters in this section directly address some clinical ethics questions in ART, and they provide frameworks that will help you think through other questions.

Discussion Questions

Chapter 5: Harris, "The Reproduction of Stratified (Assisted) Reproduction: Epidemiology, History, and Ideology in Infertility Care"
Many ART patients pay out-of-pocket. How has this history shaped the field? "Advanced maternal age" is typically considered a medical indication for ART services, so if an older patient's insurance plan covers ART services generally, it will cover hers as well. What does this fact say about "stratified reproduction"? The American Society for Reproductive Medicine (ASRM) and others are leading a campaign to pass state laws requiring private insurers to cover ART services. Do you support laws like these? Why or why not? In 2020, no state Medicaid program covered in vitro fertilization or artificial insemination, and only one state (New York) covered fertility drugs.[6] Would you support a campaign to change that? Why or why not?

Chapter 6: Gutmann Koch, "Preimplantation Genetics: Liabilities and Limitations"
Some patients do not know preimplantation genetic testing (PGT) exists. When, if ever, do you think clinicians have an ethical duty to offer PGT to patients? Is there a legal duty created by the law of informed decision-making? Are there any reasons for PGT that would lead you to decline to participate in a case? Reasons that you think your institution should refuse to do PDT?

Chapter 7: Ross, "Who Are Your Patients, and What Happens when They Disagree? Conflicts in Treating Multiple Parties Engaging in Third-Party Reproduction"
Is it possible for a doctor to ethically treat as patients both the woman donating her oocytes and the recipient she's paired with? If yes, what steps must be taken to ensure patient care for each? If no, why is this a common practice? What can physicians do to help prevent decision-making conflicts between gestational surrogates and intended parents?

Chapter 8: Klock, "Ethical Issues in Gamete Donation"
Imagine your patient is working to create a pregnancy with donated gametes, and they tell you they don't plan to tell the resulting child this fact. How would you counsel them? Federal law prohibits paying for organs: How is payment to gamete donors different from (or the same as) payment for organs? Should people paid to give gametes be called "donors"? Do you think there is such a thing as a payment that is "too high"? If yes, how do you define that number, and what are the risks of intended parents paying it?

Chapter 9: de Carvalho, Kliemchen Rodrigues, and Woodruff, "Oncofertility: Ethics and Hope After Cancer"
To what degree is fertility preservation for cancer patients targeted at medical side effects of cancer and its treatment and to what degree is it targeted at emotional or social side effects? Do the odds of success play any role in your analysis? And is this distinction of any consequence to you? How would you counsel a patient with cancer about the possibility of using an experimental procedure for possible fertility preservation? What will you do when parents want fertility preservation, but the adolescent cancer patient does not? What about the reverse situation?

Chapter 10: Brunet and Fournier, "Accessing Reproductive Technology in France: Strengths and Limits of a Model That Privileges 'Just Reproduction' Above Respect for Autonomy"

The authors analyze how ART policy in France reflects French culture and values. Apply this approach to US ART policy: What does it tell us about American culture and values? Is there anything about the French model of ART provision that you would like to see adopted in the United States? If yes why, and if no what makes the US model preferable in your opinion?

References

1. Centers for Disease Control. 2018 National Summary and Clinic Table Dataset. https://www.cdc.gov/art/artdata/index.html
2. Centers for Disease Control and Prevention, American Society for Reproductive Medicine, Society for Assisted Reproductive Technology. *2016 Assisted Reproductive Technology National Summary Report*. Atlanta, GA: US Dept of Health and Human Services; 2018.
3. MCL §722.859.
4. Centers for Disease Control and Prevention, American Society for Reproductive Medicine, Society for Assisted Reproductive Technology. *2016 Assisted Reproductive Technology National Summary Report*, 8.
5. Ibid., 53.
6. Weigel G, Ranji U, Long M, Salganicoff A. Kaiser Family Foundation Issue Brief: Coverage and Use of Fertility Services in the U.S. September 15, 2020. (https://www.kff.org/womens-health-policy/issue-brief/coverage-and-use-of-fertility-services-in-the-u-s/)

5

The Reproduction of Stratified (Assisted) Reproduction

Epidemiology, History, and Ideology in Infertility Care

Lisa H. Harris MD, PhD

I am running late in clinic, as usual. It is summer 1999, the end of my first year as a new obstetrics and gynecology faculty member. Even after almost a year, I had not figured out how to see patients within the short time period the powers-that-be gave me. The 15- or 20-minute appointment slots were rarely enough to get to know people, to find out what mattered most to them, and I chronically ran late. Today was no exception. Before heading into the next room, I glance quickly at the computer printout of my schedule, pinned to the bulletin board in the doctors' room: "New patient – infertility evaluation." I am relieved—both because I get a bit more time for new patients and because, as a resident, I had seen many patients for infertility care. I knew the work-up well, and I knew when to send patients on to reproductive endocrinologists for high-tech assisted reproductive technologies, which so often seemed to be the path for the 30- and 40-something professional women who dominated the infertility practices where I trained.

I quickly think through my infertility clinical algorithms. I knock on the door, turn the handle, and walk in. A young, maybe 20-something African American woman is seated on the chair inside. She is wearing frayed jeans, a t-shirt, and beat-up white canvas sneakers. She smiles nervously. I do a double take. I'm in the wrong room. I confirm her name. I am in the right place. I feel my face flush. Somewhere in those moments between looking at the schedule and entering the exam room, I had generated a mental picture of the patient waiting inside: she was older, white, dressed far more nicely than me, and aggravated that I was running late because she had to get back to her high-powered job somewhere. I compose myself, hope my patient didn't notice my blunder, and the visit begins.

Later that day, when the rush of patients and accompanying charting is done, I replay that moment. And I confront the reality that my idea of "infertility" (and no doubt life itself) was powerfully shaped along race and class lines.

As I describe in this chapter, there were epidemiological, historical, and, most importantly, ideological roots under my assumption, and these origins make my error understandable, though unacceptable. There is value in revisiting this moment, one that has stayed with me for nearly two decades, because it shows how stratified reproduction—the differential valuing of the fertility and childbearing of different populations—is alive and well and takes different forms at different times. Revisiting this moment may also begin to model a process for healthcare providers, especially white ones like me who benefit most from the stratification of reproduction and of all aspects of US social life, to begin the consciousness-raising required to change race and class hierarchies. While usual bioethical analyses of infertility treatment focus on the questions raised in sensational cases ("Frozen Embryo Conceived the Year After Her Mother Was Born"[1]; The Girl with Three Biological Parents"[2]), I want to consider the race and class coding of infertility as a *moral* issue because, as I'll conclude, it is a question of whose lives matter.

Epidemiological Roots of My Error

Sometimes healthcare providers engage in statistical discrimination; that is, they (we) consciously or unconsciously use probabilistic reasoning about a population-level phenomenon to make clinical decisions about individual patients. If the prevalence of infertility is highest in white women, epidemiologically speaking, it might have been understandable for me to expect to see a white person behind the door. It is not. Although fertility declines with age, the best data at the time indicated that, at any age, Black women are 1.5 to 2 times as likely to experience infertility compared to their white counterparts,[3] mirroring other reproductive health disparities, including maternal mortality, in which women of color are worse off. And, controlling for age, infertility rates *decrease* as education increases.[4] My mental image of "woman with infertility" was really flawed. Indeed, most primary care doctors mistakenly believe that infertility is primarily a problem of white professional women. In Ceballo and colleagues' study of 1,000 Michigan physicians, nearly all believed that white, highly educated Americans were most at risk of infertility.[5] Fewer than 1% correctly identified the sociodemographic predictors of infertility.

Although physicians' understanding of infertility epidemiology is remarkably poor, the expectation that a white professional woman waits behind the exam room door may be related to epidemiological patterns in care-seeking. In the United States, those most likely to access infertility care are white, married, insured, older college graduates.[4] So, from the standpoint of healthcare providers, infertility indeed appears to be a problem of older white women. Reasons for the differences in care-seeking or obtaining care undoubtedly include health insurance coverage and the related issue of income inequality in the United States. Only 16 states require private health insurance coverage of infertility treatment, and mandates vary widely in the services they require.[6] Therefore, for many people infertility care requires access to significant financial resources, resources concentrated disproportionately among white, professional Americans. State insurance mandates don't diversify the infertility patient population.[7] Less than half of state public insurance programs cover infertility diagnostic testing, and only one state requires coverage of fertility treatments like prescription medications to stimulate ovulation. None covers in vitro fertilization.[8] Since patients of color use public insurance to pay for healthcare at disproportionately higher rates than do white patients,[9] disparities in care may be related to differences in access to private health insurance coverage.

When women of color obtain care, they have usually waited longer than white women before doing so.[10] This points to the likely contribution of provider-level quality of care factors, including delays in referral for specialized care. And it may be related to patient factors: some women of color themselves internalize the idea that infertility is not something with which black women struggle. Ceballo documented that some African American women think of infertility as "a white thing," that "it didn't happen to us."[11] Ceballo's study suggested that black women carry the shame and stigma that any woman might face when she can't become pregnant, as well as the additional stigmatizing burden of feeling unlike all other black women. Both likely contribute to delays or difficulty seeking care.

Historical Origins of My Error

How, then, did infertility "become" a white, professional problem in the public imagination, when epidemiologically it is disproportionately a problem of low-income women and women of color? While there is important historical work showing that race and social class have impacted understandings of fertility and infertility throughout US history,[12] I want to focus on the decades around introduction of in vitro fertilization (IVF) in the United States in the 1980s. The rise of this new technology came at a time of immense social change, and these social contexts shaped IVF in the public imagination.

IVF worked by bypassing damaged or absent fallopian tubes and offered hope for couples for whom older treatments like hormones and sperm donation could never work. Lesley Brown was the first beneficiary of IVF treatment, giving birth to Louise in 1978. Gynecologist Patrick Steptoe and researcher John Edwards in England joined Lesley's egg with her husband's sperm, then transferred the in vitro conceived embryo to Brown's uterus.[13] Three years later, Judy Carr gave birth to Elizabeth, the first American IVF baby. Doctors Howard and Georgeanna Jones in Norfolk Virginia led the team that made her birth possible.[14] The late 1970s and beyond were years in which new, seemingly miraculous technological reproduction became newsworthy.

This period also witnessed profound private and public sphere shifts, especially for white, middle-class women who had new opportunities for reproductive autonomy. The development of the oral contraceptive pill in 1960, the legalization of contraception for all women in 1972, and the legalization of abortion in 1973 made it increasingly possible for people with access to healthcare to control the timing and number of their children. And, in the wake of Title IX's 1972 legal mandates, women experienced new educational opportunities as colleges and universities admitted more women into higher education. These opportunities in turn meant that women began to occupy new managerial and professional roles. IVF grew up with, so to speak, changing women's roles, and this turned out to have a profound effect on the technology and on ideas about infertility itself.

To be clear, the social change of the 1960s and '70s was not so much that *women* as an entire group were now working, but that particular women—white, middle-class women who after World War II had primarily private-sphere roles and depended on a husband for financial security—were now taking on higher paying professional roles that had previously been limited to white, middle-class men. Women in lower paying roles, disproportionately women of color, had, of course, worked throughout the decades in which their higher income white counterparts relied on the income of their male partners, whose opportunities and wages could independently support family life better than those of working-class men and men of color.

The combination of technologies for control of reproduction alongside new education and work opportunities for some women contributed to changes in reproductive demographics: the birthrate among American women fell by nearly half throughout the twentieth century.[15] The timing of reproduction shifted, too: women increasingly delayed childbearing. In 1970, the mean age at first birth was 21.4. It rose to 22.7 in 1980, and 23.7 in 1985.[16] And, increasingly, women delayed their first birth until their later reproductive years: first birth rate among 35- to 39-year-olds doubled between 1975 and 1985.[16] This change was driven primarily by women with college degrees, disproportionately white women.

However, fertility declines with age, and many professional women who postponed their pregnancies found that, to their shock, by the time they were ready to have children, they had difficulty conceiving. A sea change in reporting on infertility came about in the early 1980s. In February 1982, *Time* magazine introduced the term "biological clock" in its report on older women's childbearing.[17] By the mid-1980s, media reports made it appear that (white) American fertility was in a veritable crisis. Articles reported again and again that infertility was becoming a more serious problem, reaching "epidemic proportions."[18] Though demographers would later clarify that there was no new "epidemic" of infertility—meaning that infertility at any age was no greater than it had been decades earlier—media depictions created the distinct impression that there was such an epidemic.

What followed was full-out moral panic: the delayed childbearing that accompanied women's entry—largely white women's entry—into the professional workforce threatened fertility. Media messages during the 1980s urged professional women to "take control" of their reproduction in the same way that they took ownership of new career opportunities. The media told women to reevaluate their priorities and speed up reproductive timelines.[19] The fertility risks to working-class women—women by definition in the workforce, often in jobs or environments that exposed them to a range of reproductive hazards, and disproportionately women of color—were rarely discussed. The mainstream media's obsession with infertility and the "biological clock" left the distinct impression that infertility was an ailment of white professional women who delayed childbearing and needed to take control of their fertility before time ran out.

It is perhaps not surprising, then, that IVF—a newly successful technology at the time—began to be constructed in the media (and more importantly, in clinical practice) as a treatment for age-related infertility despite its origins as a treatment for tubal infertility in young women. Professional women were increasingly urged to turn to infertility specialists for help. As the media described it, IVF could solve the reproductive problems of women who had unwittingly let their career aspirations jeopardize their chance at motherhood. IVF technical advances became linked with the reproductive uncertainties brought about by women's changing life goals.

And, increasingly, women of an older reproductive age filled the appointment books in IVF clinics. Doctors began to use IVF in women over 35 and even over 40. Before 1981, patients—generally undergoing IVF in experimental protocols as there had been no US births yet—needed to be *under* age 35 and have tubal factor infertility to be eligible for IVF treatment.[20] By 1988, more than one-third (34.5%) of cycles were performed in 35- to 39-year olds; 7.5% were in women 40 or older.[21] Over the next few years, the IVF patient population continued to age; by 1990, very nearly half of IVF cycles were completed in women aged 35 or older.[22] However, success eluded most older reproductive age women. After age 40 only about 3 in 100 women could expect to take a baby home after an IVF cycle.

The technology continued to move in a direction that held promise for older women. In 1990, Dr. Mark Sauer published the first report of successful donor egg pregnancy.[23] Sauer reported in the *New England Journal of Medicine* (NEJM) that his team at the University of Southern California had treated seven women aged 40 to 44 who had undergone premature ovarian failure. He used IVF with eggs donated by younger women. Said NEJM editor Marcia Angell, "The limits on the childbearing years are now anyone's guess."[24] Sauer was subsequently "besieged" by requests from women hoping to "turn back the clock."[25]

IVF technology continued to develop in new directions that best served the needs of older, largely white, women. By the late 1990s, IVF using frozen eggs was reported, creating the possibility that women could freeze their eggs when they were young and use them later, or as *Time* reported, "stop their biological clock."[26] The potential of egg freezing to extend childbearing years was widely recognized in spite of the procedure's low success rates (around

8% in 1997). Journalists were enthusiastic about the technology. As one reporter noted, menopause might become "obsolete."[26] The IVF industry had
an enormous potential market in older professional women, who were best
positioned to afford it. Meanwhile mainstream magazines pointed to the
dearth of "healthy white babies" available for adoption, presumably by white
couples, as a reason to celebrate IVF. (Indeed, for the first decade of IVF in the
United States, no African American women or couples were photographed
or featured in magazine coverage.[27])

In the clinics, the race and socioeconomic background of patients mirrored those of media depictions—disproportionately white and economi-
cally advantaged. The first published national data on race and IVF treatment
in the late 1990s showed that black women represented 7.8% of married
reproductive-age women but underwent only 4.6% of IVF cycles.[28] Most
IVF patients had advanced degrees and earned more than $100,000/year.[29]
The fact that infertility rates were greater than 1.5 times higher for women
of color and women without a college education made these disparities even
more notable.[3] As the history of IVF shows, the technology advanced in
directions that followed the needs of the market of women who could afford it. Thus IVF—and the idea of infertility itself—became associated in the
public imagination with older, white professional women.

Ideological Origins of My Error

In 1988, the federal government's Office of Technology Assessment (OTA)
undertook an exhaustive examination of the infertility landscape in the
United States.[30] The report recognized racial and socioeconomic disparities in infertility that the media largely failed to report, namely the high, and
rising, rates of infertility among young, low-income women and women of
color. The OTA report attributed the unequal burden of infertility to the unequal burden of sexually transmitted infections (STIs) and pelvic inflamma-
tory disease (PID): whereas STIs were responsible for about 20% of infertility
nationally, in low-income women and women of color it was thought to be
responsible for as much as 50%. The OTA report described STIs as hazards of
"urban living," which was perhaps a euphemistic way of saying that they were
(and are) hazards of economic, educational, and healthcare inequalities.[30]
The good news might have been that STIs and PID caused tubal infertility,
precisely the kind of infertility IVF was designed to treat and in which success

rates were highest. In other words, low-income women and women of color would have benefitted from IVF in ways that many of the older women who did access IVF could not.

However, there was no media panic about the threats to childbearing of lower wage working women, disproportionately women of color. In these groups, of course, childbearing and hard work had never been framed as in conflict. Only one journalist, Lewis Lord, writing for *US News and World Report* in 1987, noted, "Despite its image as a yuppie woe, infertility occurs one-and-a-half times more often among blacks than among whites and is most common among high-school dropouts."[31] Besides that story and a short paragraph in *Jet* in 1984 on the difficulty of coming to grips with not having biological children,[32] the infertility of women of color and racial and socioeconomic disparities in infertility rates were neglected in nearly all media accounts. In a sea of reporting on infertility that included well over 400 newspaper and magazine articles in the 1980s in major national publications, including some targeting black readers specifically, the reproductive health needs of women of color and low-income women were almost never considered and certainly not their difficulties accessing infertility care or their potential benefit from IVF treatment. But they were about to become connected to it in paradoxical and troubling ways.

The harder IVF doctors worked to meet the reproductive needs of women who made it to their offices, the more new and previously unimagined clinical and ethical dilemmas arose. Over the next decade, as women in their late 40s, then 50s, and even 60s began to use donor egg IVF technology to become pregnant, many critics questioned if childbearing at such ages was appropriate. And at that time, media accounts began to sound a distinctly new theme: older women were the most fit parents. They were, reports offered, exceptionally well-equipped both emotionally and financially to have children. Children of older mothers, it was argued, "reap the benefits of having been born to parents who are clear and focused."[33] Babies of postmenopausal women "will be greatly cherished in a world where many children are not, and where many young women have babies with scarcely a thought."[34] Several commentators suggested that older childbearing was particularly desirable when compared to that of adolescents or girls and of women with substance use disorders: "Mature mothers make good mothers, especially in contrast to a child-parent of fifteen."[35] Said another older mother, "Of course, a child born to a responsible mother in her sixties will get a better start in life than the child of an eighteen-year-old crack cocaine addict."[35] The racialized undertones of these statements were unmistakable. As legal scholar Dorothy Roberts and others have shown, rhetoric of "crack babies" and "welfare queens" that proliferated at this time—and the social policies of coercive contraception, criminalization of pregnant women's behavior, and so-called welfare reform that accompanied it—denigrated and disavowed the motherhood of low-income women, especially women of color.

Social class references lay between the lines of these arguments as well: a professor who wrote about her difficulties conceiving contrasted the great lengths to which she and her husband went to achieve pregnancy to the "thousands of couples who are illiterate or poor or unwilling to care for their children" yet who "conceive babies regularly" with ease.[36] Such invidious comparisons conflated class position with parenting ability and commitment, or perhaps even with love for a child. IVF in older women provided a new opportunity to reveal veiled public anxiety not just about women who had difficulty becoming pregnant, but also about women who appeared to become pregnant without difficulty. And thus—as has been the case throughout US history—an ideology of stratified reproduction was reinforced as IVF technology grew. That is, media discussions of infertility and IVF came to reveal a national ethos regarding whose reproduction was prized and valued in the United States and whose was demonized and feared.

Or rather, IVF offered a new window on old ideology. Stratified experiences of reproduction have been documented throughout US history.[37] In the United States, the reproduction of white middle-class or affluent people has always been valued by those with the greatest power and resources, and the reproduction of poor and working-class white women and women of color has not and is even seen as a threat to US social fabric. As scholar Taida Wolfe and I have argued, "no matter where one 'biopsies' US history, there is evidence of preoccupation with the issue of who is reproducing and who is not, and formal and informal policies to limit the reproduction of some or encourage the reproduction of others."[38] It was true during black slavery when white slave owners determined the meanings of pregnancy based on its economic impact on planation life: they treated it as a liability before the close of the slave trade, but an asset after, when it became the only way to increase slave holdings. Stratified reproduction was evident during the period in which Native children were taken from their families to off-reservation boarding schools to "civilize" them. And it was true throughout the 1900s, when programs of coercive, compulsory sterilization left many poor women, disabled women, Latinas, and African American women permanently sterilized without their knowledge or consent. The triaging of white, older, professional woman to IVF—a technology which in its original forms was unlikely to help them—is another face of stratified reproduction.

Reproduction has powerful social meanings, about who "belongs" and who does not. The story of IVF provides one more piece of evidence that an ideology of stratified reproduction takes different forms at different times. Though it is easiest to see stratified reproduction when the fertility and child-bearing of a disadvantaged group is unjustly limited, it can also take the form of the fertility of an advantaged group being promoted or prized, as is the case here. The story of IVF adds an additional element, however: *IVF technology itself* shifted in ways that were responsive to both ideological and market needs. IVF was developed to bypass blocked, damaged, or absent fallopian tubes, a problem more common in young, low-income women and women of color. But the technology shifted to meet the needs of those whose reproductive needs mattered most to those in the position to create policy, practice, and conduct research. And importantly, it shifted to match the needs of the people who could pay for it.

Nothing I've said here diminishes the pain of the lived experience of infertility in women who did access IVF care, their joy when the technology succeeded, their immense pain when it did not, and the compassion of doctors who cared for them and who advocated for the insurance coverage we have, limited as it is. My point here is that the lived experience of women who could not access infertility care was neglected; their experiences in effect did not register as important. Indeed, if low-income black (reproductive) lives mattered, perhaps IVF care would have moved in a different direction in the 1980s and 1990s—toward lower cost, natural cycle IVF, for example, and not donor egg and egg freezing technologies using wildly expensive ovarian stimulation drugs, which were largely out of reach for poor women. The course of IVF technology was not predetermined and was not an inevitable product of its inherent technical details. Rather, its course reflected a range of social inequalities and priorities.

But, of course, why *wouldn't* reproduction be stratified when the rest of life is? The question of whose lives matter is brought to life particularly vividly when, in the face of a deep desire to have a child, some will have assistance to do so and some will not. IVF reproduces lives, so access to IVF technology shows, quite literally, that some people's lives matter and other people's don't. IVF reproduces stratified reproduction itself. This, to me, is the central ethical issue in IVF care.

My patient 20 years ago ultimately did not need IVF. In fact, she did not want to become pregnant, but worried she might be infertile because she didn't become pregnant after a single episode of unprotected sex. Our conversation and a few basic tests proved reassuring. I still wonder if she picked up my blunder. And I also wonder why an episode of unprotected sex that didn't result in pregnancy caused her to make a doctor's appointment when so many other people would have simply breathed a sigh of relief. Had she also internalized stereotypes about fertility and infertility, in this case that she should be able to become pregnant exceedingly easily? I did not have the words or insight at that moment to ask either question. However, that encounter stayed with me and started a research journey into the history of IVF, some of which is reflected here, as well as a personal journey into understanding how I contribute to the racial organization of medicine and life and my role in righting reproductive injustices and undoing white privilege.

Social life and medical care co-create each other; that is, gender, race, and social class intersect to produce IVF care, and, in turn, IVF technology reinforces and reinvigorates the social world that created it. That moment of walking into the exam room is evidence of the social construction of bodies, health, illness, and medical care and of the way in which unconscious bias seeps into everything. It is, and ought to remain, my everyday struggle to dismantle the gender, race, and social class inequalities expressed routinely in medical care.

Acknowledgments

The author would like to thank Meghan Seewald, Celina Doria, Liza Fuentes, and Phyllis Watts, as well as the Editors, for helpful comments on an earlier draft.

References

1. CNN. 2017. https://www.cnn.com/2017/12/19/health/snowbaby-oldest-embryo-bn/index.html September 1, 2014.
2. BBC. https://www.bbc.com/news/magazine-28986843
3. Stephen EH, Chandra A. Declining estimates of infertility in the United States: 1982–2002. *Fertil Steril* 2006;86:516–23.

4. Chandra A, Copen C, Stephen EH. Infertility service use in the United States: Data from the National Survey of Family Growth, 1982–2010. *Nat Health Stat Rep.* 2014 Jan 22;73.

5. Ceballo R, Abbey A, Schooler D. Perceptions of women's infertility: What do doctor's see? *Fertil Steril.* 2010 Mar 1;93(4):1066–73.

6. National Conference of State Legislatures. State laws related to insurance coverage for infertility treatment. 2018 Apr. http://www.ncsl.org/research/health/insurance-coverage-for-infertility-laws.aspx

7. Schmidt L. Effects of infertility insurance mandates on fertility. *J Health Econ.* 2007 May;26(3):431–46.

8. Weigel G, Ranji U, Long M, Salganicoff A. Kaiser Family Foundation Issue Brief: Coverage and Use of Fertility Services in the U.S. September 15, 2020. https://www.kff.org/womens-health-policy/issue-brief/coverage-and-use-of-fertility-services-in-the-u-s/

9. Kaiser Family Foundation. Health coverage by race and ethnicity: The potential impact of the Affordable Care Act. 2013 Mar. https://www.kff.org/racial-equity-and-health-policy/issue-brief/health-coverage-by-race-and-ethnicity-the-potential-impact-of-the-affordable-care-act/

10. Chin HB, Howards P, Kramer M, Mertens A, Spencer J. Racial disparities in seeking care for help getting pregnant. *Paediatr Perinat Epidemiol.* 2015 Sep;29(5):416–25.

11. Ceballo R. "The only black woman walking the face of the earth who can't have a baby": Two women's stories. In Romero M, Stewart AJ, eds., *Women's Untold Stories: Breaking Silence, Talking Back, Voicing Complexity.* New York: Routledge; 1999: 12.

12. May ET. *Barren in the Promised Land: Childless Americans and the pursuit of Happiness.* New York: Basic Books; 1995.

13. Wang J, Sauer M. In vitro fertilization (IVF): A review of 3 decades of clinical innovation and technological advancement. *Ther Clin Risk Manag.* 2006 Dec;2(4):355–64.

14. Jones H. The use of controlled ovarian hyperstimulation (COH) in clinical in vitro fertilization: The role of Georgeanna Seegar Jones. *Fertil Steril.* 2008 Nov;90(5):1–3.

15. The birthrate fell from thirty births per thousand people in 1910 to sixteen births per thousand people in 1980. See Michigan Department of Community Health. Live births and crude birth rates—Michigan and United States Residents, 1900–2011, http://www.mdch.state.mi.us/pha/osr/natality/tab1.1.asp

16. The birthrate in women aged 35–39 rose from 19.8 per 1,000 in 1975 to 39.3 per 1,000 in 1985. Stephanie J. Ventura et al. *Trends in pregnancies and pregnancy rates by outcome: Estimates for the United States, 1976–1996.* Series 21: Data from the National Vital Statistics System, No. 56. Hyattsville, MD: National Center for Health Statistics; 2000.

17. Cocks J. The new Baby Bloom. *Time,* 1982 Feb 22:52–7.

18. Isaacs F. High-tech pregnancies. *Good Housekeeping.* 1986 Feb:81. Author attributes figure to the American Fertility Society.

19. Podolsky, "Having Babies Past 40," 105. U.S. News & World Report. 1990;109(17):105–10.

20. Acosta A, Andrews MC, Jones GS et al. The indications for in vitro fertilization. *Virginia Med.* 1986 Apr;113:217.

21. Medical Research International and Society for Assisted Reproductive Technology. In vitro fertilization-embryo transfer (IVF-ET) in the United States: 1988 results

from the National IVF-ET Registry. *Fertil Steril.* 1990 Jan;53(1):13–20. Age break-down of patients was not provided in 1985–1987. "Cycles" here means fresh (rather than frozen) embryo, non-donor egg cycles. In 1988, breakdowns are provided for the first time for those patients undergoing fresh, non-donor IVF cycles, as it was be-coming more and more apparent that age might be related to success rates.

22. Medical Research International and Society for Assisted Reproductive Technology. In vitro fertilization–embryo transfer (IVF-ET) in the United States: 1990. *Fertil Steril.* 1992 Jan;57(1):15–24. Age breakdowns were not provided in the 1991 report. See also: In vitro fertilization–embryo transfer (IVF-ET) in the United States: 1989. *Fertil Steril.* 1991 Jan;55(1):14–22; In vitro fertilization–embryo transfer (IVF-ET) in the United States: 1988. *Fertil Steril.* 1990 Jan;53(1):13–20. Absolute numbers of cycles were calculated by multiplying the total number of cycles done that year by the fraction of cycles done in patients in each age group. In 1988, the total number of fresh, non-donor cycles was 13,647. Therefore 7,901 cycles (57.9%) were done in patients <35 years, 4,708 cycles (34.5%) in 35- to 39-year-olds, and 1,023 cycles (7.5%) in women ≥40. In 1989, 18,211 fresh non-donor cycles were done: 10,380 (57%) in patients <35 years, 6,319 (34.7%) in 35- to 39-year-olds, and 1,511 (8.3%) in women ≥40. In 1990, a total of 19,079 fresh, non-donor cycles were done: 9,215 (48.3%) were in women <35, which represents a decline of 11% in absolute number of cycles in this age group; 7,307 (38.3%) were in women 35–39 years old, a jump of 15.6%. Finally, 2,556 cycles (13.4%) were done in women ≥40, a jump of 69% from the previous year.

23. Sauer MV, Paulson RJ, Lobo RA. A preliminary report on oocyte donation extending reproductive potential to women over 40. *N Engl J Med.* 1990;323(17):1157–60.

24. Angell M. New ways to get pregnant. *N Engl J Med.* 1990;323(17):1200–2. Quoted in Making babies after menopause: A stunning new success. *Newsweek.* 1990 Nov 5:75.

25. Kolata G. Giving older women a shot at motherhood. *New York Times.* 1990 Oct 28:E4.

26. Gorman C. How old is too old? *Time.* 1991 Sep 30:62.

27. Harris LH. *Challenging Conception: A Clinical and Cultural History of In Vitro Fertilization in the United States.* PhD dissertation. University of Michigan, Ann Arbor, 2006.

28. Seifer DB, Frazier LM, Grainger DA. Disparity in assisted reproductive technologies outcomes in black women compared with white women. *Fertil Steril.* 2008;90:1701–10. Data were limited by the fact that fewer than half of clinics (48.4%) reporting their data to the Society for Assisted Reproductive Technology and the Centers for Disease control reliably included data on patient race/ethnicity.

29. Jain T, Hornstein MD. Disparities in access to infertility services in a state with man-dated insurance coverage. *Fertil Steril.* 2005;84:221–3.

30. US Congress, Office of Technology Assessment. *Infertility: Medical and Social Choices,* OTA-BA-358 Washington, DC: US Government Printing Office; 1988 May.

31. Lord L. Desperately seeking baby. *US News World Rep.* 1987 Oct 5:59. See also Mosher WD, Pratt WF. *Fecundity and Infertility in the United States, 1965–1982.* Advance Data No. 104. Hyattsville, MD: National Center for Health Statistics; 1985 Feb 11.

32. Couples may have trouble adjusting to infertility. *Jet.* 1984 Oct 29.

33. Kolata G. Childbirth at 63 says what about life? *New York Times.* 1997 Apr 27.

34. Beck M, Hager M, Wingert P, et al. How far should we push mother nature? *Newsweek.* 1994;54.
35. Wall JM. A time to be born. *Christian Century.* 1997 May 14:468.
36. Frank E. The struggle to have a child. *New York Times.* 1985 Apr 28:CN 26.
37. Roberts D. *Killing the Black Body—Race, Reproduction and the Meaning of Liberty.* New York: Random House; 1997.
38. Harris LH, Wolfe T. Stratified reproduction, family planning care and the double edge of history. *Curr Opin Obstet Gynecol.* 2014 Dec;26(6):539–44.

6

Preimplantation Genetics

Liabilities and Limitations

Valerie Gutmann Koch JD

Assisted reproduction and emerging technologies and interventions offer an increasing range of choices to would-be parents. This chapter addresses the various uses and ethical implications of preimplantation genetic testing (PGT), which enables the screening and selection of embryos for chromosomal abnormalities and genetic traits before implantation.[1] It then addresses the topic of liability as it applies to PGT, highlighting the potential reliance on wrongful life claims to remedy harms that may occur as a result of using such testing. In doing so, the chapter endeavors to provide a foundation for healthcare providers who provide PGT regarding key potential liabilities and ethical considerations.

There are two major types of ethical objections to PGT. The first is a wholesale objection to using the technology at all due to the fact that it almost invariably leads to the intentional destruction of human embryos. Consequently, this objection is often based on the moral status of embryos and arguments that no embryo should be discarded. The second type of ethical objection is to the act of selecting particular embryos based on genetic testing. This chapter focuses on this second type of objection, which hinges on the question of *why* individuals are seeking to use the technology. Importantly, US law does not place restrictions on the use of PGT, and therefore, legally, the technology could presumably be used for almost any purpose imagined.

The Centers for Disease Control and Prevention (CDC) asks that all clinics providing in vitro fertilization (IVF) report pregnancy success rates annually to the web-based National Assisted Reproductive Technology (ART) Surveillance System, but reporting of PGT use and outcomes is not required. According to estimates, between 2011 and 2012, 9% of the approximately 107,000 IVF cycles performed utilized PGT. A total of 55.6% of these were performed to screen for chromosomal abnormalities, 15.3% for genetic testing (PGT genetic), and 29.1% for "other reasons."[2] While any of these uses of PGT are potentially accessible to would-be parents, because of a dearth of reporting requirements in the United States, it is difficult to determine exactly how and why it is being used.

PGT is often sought when the intended parents hope to lower the risk of transmitting medical conditions caused by single-gene mutations—particularly childhood diseases—to offspring. Thus, PGT may be used to rule out implantation of embryos with devastating diseases that manifest in infancy or childhood. In many cases, IVF combined with PGT is an alternative to prenatal testing—and subsequent pregnancy termination—for would-be parents seeking to avoid having a child with these diseases.

The use of PGT for diseases that manifest later in life, if at all, is more ethically contentious. Some distinguish between screening for Mendelian conditions and "susceptibility" conditions.[3] In light of emerging treatments, the promise of future cures, and the inconclusive predictive nature of tests, PGT for diseases that may not present themselves for many decades (or at all) necessitates increased ethical scrutiny. In 2013, the ethics committee of the American Society for Reproductive Medicine (ASRM) issued its guidance for use of PGT for adult-onset conditions. It concluded that PGT is ethically justifiable when the condition is serious and when there are no known interventions for the condition, or the available interventions are either inadequately effective or significantly burdensome.[4] Furthermore, it opined that, for conditions that are less serious or of lower penetrance, PGT for adult-onset conditions is ethically acceptable as a matter of reproductive liberty. It should be discouraged, however, if the risks of PGT are more than merely speculative.

Another potential—although relatively infrequent—use of PGT is for the creation of so-called savior siblings. In such cases, families have an already-born child with a congenital or acquired bone marrow disease who needs a stem cell transplant to live.[5] Ethicists have expressed concern about commodification or exploitation of a future-born child, treating a child as means to an end, and the imposition of the risks of IVF, embryo biopsy, and later possible intrusive medical interventions on a healthy child for the benefit of someone else.[6] Others have countered that the child would be no less loved or cared for due to the circumstances of their birth.[7]

Increasingly, PGT may be used for "nontherapeutic" purposes, including sex selection[8] and (in the future) to select for genetic predispositions to nonmedical traits such as hair color, eye color, and intelligence.[9] Although the US population does not appear to prefer one sex over the other,[10] many worry that sex selection could lead to great disparities in the sex ratio of the population in other countries, such as China and India.[11] Others express concern that sex selection will further emphasize and reinforce archaic gender expectations.[12] The use of PGT to select for (or against) other "nontherapeutic" traits raises the specter of eugenics, concerns about "designer" children, and questions of justice and equality.

Finally, PGT may be used to select *for* certain traits that society generally views as undesirable. In such cases, parents who themselves often have the traits they are seeking for their future child (e.g., deafness or achondroplasia) seek to transfer embryos that test positive for those same traits so that the child may be a member of the parents' community and culture.[13]

Currently, there are no consistent liability rules specific to the provision of (or the failure to provide) preimplantation testing. In light of the dearth of statutory law and regulations, what happens when something goes wrong? Despite guidance from ASRM to the contrary,[14] a 2008 study of US fertility clinics found that only a little more than one in five clinics report errors in diagnosing, labeling, and handling donor samples and embryos for implantation.[15]

However, the harms that arise from the use of preimplantation testing that might lead to legal liability may be somewhat unique and require special consideration. Unlike other assisted reproductive technologies and interventions, PGT occurs *after* conception but *before* implantation, and thus one need not address harms that occur when either a pregnancy occurs but was unwanted or when a pregnancy is sought but is not attained.[16]

There are several categories of errors or wrongs that can occur in the provision of preimplantation testing, including the negligent testing, selection, and implantation of IVF embryos. Frequently, liability occurs due to a provider's failure to detect or warn of the potential for genetic anomaly and the resultant birth of a child with that anomaly. Parents might claim that the provider failed to properly inform them of (1) the inherent errors associated with the PGT process, (2) a facility's minimal experience in performing PGT, or (3) PGT as a treatment option.[17] Liability can occur when risks are not properly communicated or where the wrong embryo is implanted. Conversely, it is possible that, when parents seek to have a child with a certain (at least socially) anomalous trait and the child is born without that trait, the parents will seek compensation.

When wrongs occur, there may be significant medical, psychological, and economic implications for those individuals who sought preimplantation testing to avoid a genetic disease or to improve the chance of achieving pregnancy. Those who are harmed may rely on a number of types of claims against facilities and physicians—most of which are based in tort law, or civil (private) law (rather than criminal law). Many of these cases are settled before they ever see the inside of a courtroom, so there is scant data on how often these cases are brought and for how much they are settled. Most claims that have or can be brought by one party against another with respect to PGT are negligence claims—the failure to use reasonable care. In other words, individuals allege that they were injured or harmed due to the negligent testing, selection, and implantation of IVF embryos.[18] Plaintiffs seeking to recover in these negligence cases typically rely on one of three types of claims: informed consent claims, wrongful birth claims, and wrongful life claims. Each will be considered in turn.

Informed consent claims are based on the failure of healthcare providers to disclose information regarding medical options. In the case of PGT, such legal claims may include the failure to disclose the risk of fetal abnormality, birth defects, or even undesirable traits in the resulting child.

In one case, a couple alleged that IVF providers at Columbia University and Columbia-Presbyterian Medical Center failed to conduct a preimplantation genetic test to ascertain whether the donor egg had genetic diseases. The couple's child was born with cystic fibrosis (CF). The couple alleged that they were told that the donor did not have a history of mental illness or genetic diseases and that they were never given information about the potential for CF. The New York Court stated that the parents would be permitted to "vigorously pursue recovery" due to the defendant's failure to follow the standard of care in screening for CF, thus allowing the plaintiffs to seek monetary damages resulting from caring for a child with CF. The parties later settled for $1.3 million before trial.[19]

In a similar case, parents sued an IVF clinic for failure to inform them of the option for PGT. After their child was born with Down syndrome, the South Carolina couple sued the fertility clinic in Charlotte, North Carolina, that provided the IVF services, alleging that the clinic's failure to offer IVF patients the option of preimplantation genetic diagnosis led to "substantial financial expenses." They claimed that they should have been informed of the option for preimplantation genetic diagnosis before their initial IVF cycle.

The case was never decided on the merits but was dismissed on procedural grounds (lack of jurisdiction).[20]

Wrongful birth claims arise when parents object to the birth of an unwanted or unplanned child. In such cases, the parents allege that the physician failed to warn them of the risk of conceiving or giving birth to a child with a serious genetic disorder, arguing that the birth of an ill or disabled child caused the parents harm.[21] In these cases, parents recover from the harm *they* experience from the healthcare providers' negligence, which resulted in the birth of an unwanted or disabled child. More than half of states permit wrongful birth actions.[22] However, because wrongful birth claims are intended to help the parents be compensated for their injury, damages in these types of cases are limited to the cost of raising the child until the age of majority.[23]

As an example of a wrongful birth case, a jury awarded $50 million—the largest individual award in Washington state history—to a couple whose son was born with "unbalanced chromosome translocation" leading to profound mental and physical disabilities. The parents brought a wrongful birth case against the medical center and lab, alleging that the lab missed the translocation because the medical center mishandled the genetic test and failed to send vital information to the lab. The couple claimed that, had they known of the genetic defect, they would have ended the pregnancy.[24]

In another case, a couple underwent IVF and preimplantation genetic diagnosis with the sole intention of avoiding having a child with cystic fibrosis (CF). The parents were known carriers of CF. After IVF of 10 eggs by New York University (NYU) personnel, biopsies of each embryo were sent to Genesis Genetics, a company that specializes in providing preimplantation genetic diagnosis laboratory services, to be tested. The report faxed to the NYU IVF facility identified two embryos, those numbered 8 and 10, as "Carrier maternal—OK to transfer." Embryologists and an endocrinologist at NYU instead substituted embryo number 7, which had been identified as "Carrier at worst," for embryo 10. The NYU defendants subsequently implanted embryo 7. Two weeks after their child's birth, the daughter was diagnosed with CF.

The couple alleged that NYU IVF facilities and Genesis Genetics were negligent in their embryo screening program. The Grossbaums sought monetary damages for emotional distress, cost and expenses of medical care, and continuing care for the child after the age of majority. The court did not decide the factual merits of the case as it resolved the case on procedural grounds (the couple filed their claim too late—outside the statute of limitations for medical malpractice claims in New York).[25]

Finally, wrongful life claims are those in which the child (as represented by the child's parents or a guardian) alleges that he or she would have been better off never having lived at all, and, but for the physician's (or parents') negligence, would not in fact have lived. Wrongful life claims are not about whether, but for the defendant's negligence, the child would have had a healthy, unimpaired life; instead, the claim is that without the doctor or parents' negligence, the child never would have existed.[26] All but three states (California, Washington and New Jersey) refuse to recognize this cause of action.[27] And even in those jurisdictions, recovery has been limited to the extraordinary medical and educational expenses associated with the impairment.

In cases where the child was born with an impairment that was detectable *during* pregnancy wrongful life claims have been relatively easily dismissed,[28] particularly because there is no legal precedent for holding a woman liable for failing to terminate a pregnancy, even after learning that the child would be born with a devastating disease. However, wrongful life claims may be more accessible in cases in which would-be parents seek PGT because those cases generally do not implicate the right to seek a legal abortion. Rather, errors that occur during PGT generally occur before the embryo is implanted, and therefore such cases do not elicit arguments concerning a woman's ability to make decisions during a pregnancy.[29]

However, even in the context of PGT, wrongful life cases are rarely allowed. For example, in 2000, Thomas Doolan, a minor child, attempted to bring a wrongful life claim. His parents were both carriers of the gene for CF. They had already had a child with the disease and they underwent IVF with PGT solely for the purpose of avoiding having another child with CF. Despite these efforts, Thomas was born with CF. He sued the IVF providers for wrongful life, arguing that such a claim is appropriate in the context of preimplantation testing.[30] The court held that the child could not bring such a claim, noting that the same "fundamental problem of logic" existed as with other previous wrongful life cases: there was no way the infant "could ever have been born without" the disease.[31]

There are a number of arguments against allowing such wrongful life claims. First, scholars and courts have raised slippery slope concerns. For example, an Illinois court worried that finding for the son in his wrongful life suit against his father would encourage others to "seek damages for being born of a certain color, another because of race; one for being born with a hereditary disease, another for inheriting unfortunate family characteristics; one for being born into a large and destitute family, another because a parent has an unsavory reputation."[32]

Second, because negligence claims require a duty between the person causing the harm and the person harmed, it can be quite unclear to whom the duty of care is owed. Is it owed by the physician or parent to the not-yet-implanted embryo? Do prospective children have rights such that parents and physicians owe them a duty of care? This raises the inherent problem with considering the embryo a legal "person" or prospective "person"; such a designation would have enormous implications for other areas of the law where embryos are not given the same legal status as a born person.[33]

Third, because a plaintiff must demonstrate that the harm resulted in damages in order to prevail on a tort claim, wrongful life claims imply that life itself can be considered an injury. As the Illinois Supreme Court has stated, public policy mandates against the "judgment that an individual life is so wretched that one would have been better off not to exist."[34] The disability rights community, in particular, has countered that considering life itself to be an injury demonstrates unacceptable discrimination against existing individuals with disabilities.[35] These arguments currently arise in the context of prenatal testing, particularly in the context of screening for Down syndrome, which is the standard of care.

In tort law generally, damages (compensation for loss or injury) are intended to return the injured individual to the position he or she would have been in had the harm not occurred. Proof of actual injury in typical negligence claims is difficult enough. But, in wrongful life cases, the question arises of how to calculate the value of an individual's own existence since that very existence is the wrong being claimed.[36] The question of how to calculate the value of the injury if the injury is life itself also implicates the now-famous non-identity problem, in which Derek Parfit reasoned that there is no way to calculate the value of the injury since the resulting child would not exist but for the actions of the parents and healthcare providers.[37] Even those few courts that have recognized wrongful life claims limit damages to recovery of extraordinary medical expenses and not damages for the loss of enjoyment of life, including the child's diminished childhood.[38]

Forbidding wrongful life claims may, instinctually, seem like the correct response: one should not be able to claim she should not have been born because she was born with the "wrong" color eyes or height, or—in the case where parents sought to select *for* certain "undesirable" traits like deafness—was born with full hearing. But what about the hypothetical case where PGT is sought to produce a savior sibling, but because it was negligently performed resulted in the birth of an infant with an HLA type which does not match the older sibling? Might the older sibling have a cause of action? If so, how would the value of that injury be calculated?

Although this chapter is focused on PGT—a technology already available to would-be parents—considerations of genetic modification are not just the stuff of science fiction.[39] Scholars have raised the question of whether the arguments regarding the non-identity problem would similarly apply to cases involving genetic modification.[40] In 2017, a panel of the National Academy of Sciences recommended that germline modification of human beings be permitted in the future in certain narrow circumstances to prevent the birth of children with a "serious disease or condition," but only with "stringent oversight."[41] If this report is an indication of the future of reproductive interventions, questions of liability will inevitably arise when things go wrong. And, as some scholars have noted, the argument that the non-identity problem precludes recovery for wrongful life when PGT is used would not apply when addressing questions involving preimplantation genetic modification, thus further complicating the application of the non-identity problem to modern technology.[42]

Although, legally, preimplantation genetic diagnosis could presumably be used for almost any purpose, negligence in the provision of PGT could expose providers to liability. Providers of PGT would therefore be wise to be aware of—and attempt to avoid—actions that might result in allegations of failure to obtain informed consent or in wrongful birth and wrongful life claims. In particular, while wrongful life claims are generally not recognized by the courts, it is worth considering how these claims might be supported in the context of harms that arise during PGT and new medical innovations.

In addition to providing care that meets the standard of care (thereby avoiding potential legal liability), providers would also be well-served to consider how liability rules affect both their own actions as well as parental decision-making. These rules influence social outcomes, and thus, in offering PGT to would-be parents, institutions and providers should contemplate a number of ethical issues. For example, how does society approach issues of disability? Might there be societal duties to provide (or, conversely, not provide) preimplantation diagnosis? Is the pursuit of genetic enhancement even acceptable—and if so, under what conditions?

References

1. After a harvested egg is fertilized in vitro, a single cell is removed from the days-old embryo, which is tested for genetic or chromosomal abnormalities. Certain embryo(s) are then chosen to be transferred to the woman's uterus to implant. In 2008, PGT was used in almost 4% of all IVF cycles. Baruch S, Kaufman DJ, Hudson KL. Preimplantation genetic screening: A survey of in vitro fertilization clinics. *Genet Med.* 2008;10:685–90. The first established pregnancies utilizing PGT were reported in 1990. Handyside AH, Kontogianni EH, Hardy K, Winston RM. Pregnancies from biopsied human preimplantation embryos sexed by Y-specific DNA amplification. *Nature.* 1990;344(6268):768–70.

2. Chang J, Boulet SL, Jeng G, et al. Outcomes of in vitro fertilization with preimplantation genetic diagnosis: An analysis of the United States assisted reproductive technology surveillance data, 2011–2012. *Fertil Steril.* 2016;105(2):394–400.

3. Robertson JA. Extending preimplantation genetic diagnosis: The ethical debate: ethical issues in new uses of preimplantation genetic diagnosis. *Human Reprod.* 2003;18(3):465–71. For example, with diseases such as Huntington's disease, the HTT mutation is an effective "on/off" switch, meaning the resulting child will eventually develop the devastating disease as an adult.

4. Ethics Committee of the American Society for Reproductive Medicine. Use of preimplantation genetic diagnosis for serious adult onset conditions: A committee opinion. *Fertil Steril.* 2013;100:54–7.

5. In such cases, the parents undergo IVF and PGT for human leukocyte antigen (HLA) typing in order to have another child who would serve as a source of stem cells, either obtained from that child's umbilical cord blood or bone marrow.

6. Lai ATY. To be or not to be my sister's keeper?: A revised legal framework safeguarding savior siblings' welfare. *J Leg Med.* 2011;32:261–93.

7. Robertson. Extending preimplantation genetic diagnosis. John Robertson has stated that, in fact, that because the child's "birth might save the life of an existing, loved child," it might "only increase its specialness." Moreover, couples have children for all sorts of reasons—including saving a marriage, because their peers are doing so, or because their contraception failed.

8. Baruch S, Kaufman D, Hudson KL. Genetic testing of embryos: Practices and perspectives of US in vitro fertilization clinics. *Fertil Steril.* 2008;89(5):1053–8. This study found that 42% of IVF-PGT clinics used these technologies for nonmedical sex selection. However, only 41% of those clinics reported that they would provide the service for a second or subsequent child and not for a first-born child.

9. Regalado A. Eugenics 2.0: We're at the dawn of choosing embryos by health, height, and more. *MIT Tech Rev.* 2017 Nov 1, https://www.technologyreview.com/s/609204/eugenics-20-were-at-the-dawn-of-choosing-embryos-by-health-height-and-more/. Although PGS for sex discernment may be used to test for single-gene diseases that may only present in one sex (e.g., X-linked diseases), it is considered "nontherapeutic" when used for family balancing. Vacco LA. Preimplantation genetic diagnosis: From

preventing genetic disease to customizing children. Can the technology be regulated based on the parents' intent? *St. Louis U L J.* 2005;49:1181–228.

10. Baruch S. Preimplantation genetic diagnosis and parental preferences: Beyond deadly disease. *Hous J Health & Pol'y.* 2008;8(2);245–70.

11. Bumgarner A. A right to choose?: Sex selection in the international context. *Duke J Gender L & Pol'y.* 2007;14:1289–1309.

12. Robertson JA, Hickman T. Should PGD be used for elective gender selection? *Contemporary OB/GYN.* 2013 Jul 1, http://contemporaryobgyn.modernmedicine. com/contemporary-obgyn/content/tags/american-society-reproductive-medicine/ should-pgd-be-used-elective-g?page=full; Daar JE. ART and the search for perfectionism: On selecting gender, genes, and gametes. *J Gender Race & Just.* 2005;9:241.

13. King JS. Duty to the unborn: A response to Smolensky. *Hastings L J.* 2008;60:377–96; Sanghavi DM, Wanting babies like themselves, some parents choose genetic defects. *New York Times.* 2006 Dec 5. In many such instances, the trait is considered an "identity" rather than a medical illness that should be avoided, treated, or cured.

14. Ethics Committee of the American Society for Reproductive Medicine. Disclosure of medical errors involving gametes and embryos: An ethics committee opinion. *Fertil Steril.* 2016;106(1):59–63.

15. Baruch, Kaufman, Hudson. Preimplantation genetic screening; 21% of IVF-PGT clinics reported that they had been aware of inconsistencies between the results of genetic analysis of embryos and later genetic testing.

16. Fox D. Reproductive negligence. *Columbia L Rev.* 2017;117(1):149–234. Dov Fox refers to harms that occur at the stage after conception and before implantation as "confounded reproduction," meaning that a desired pregnancy and birth will occur, but that the fetus or baby has traits not intended due to use of assisted reproduction. Besides PGT gone awry, Professor Fox also uses "confounded reproduction" to refer to situations where eggs are fertilized with the wrong sperm or where embryos are implanted into the wrong uterus.

17. Amagwula BS, Chang PL, Hossain A, et al. Preimplantation genetic diagnosis: A systematic review of litigation in the face of new technology. *Fertil Steril.* 2012;98:1277–82.

18. To prevail on a negligence claim, the plaintiff must prove four elements: that the defendant owed a duty to the plaintiff, that the defendant breached that duty, that that breach caused harm (causation), and that the harm resulted in damages.

19. *Paretta v. Medical Offices for Human Reproduction*, 195 Misc. 2d 568 (N.Y. Sup. Ct. 2003).

20. *Coggeshall v. Reproductive Endocrine Associates*, 376 S.C. 12 (2007).

21. Botkin JR. Prenatal diagnosis and the selection of children. *Fla State Univ Law Rev.* 2003;30:265.

22. Rebouché R, Rothenberg K. Mixed messages: The intersection of prenatal genetic testing and abortion. *How L Rev.* 2012;55:983. While such damages may appear quite comprehensive, they are still limited; they do not address an individual's ability to choose whether to continue (or, in the case of PGT, even start) a pregnancy. More intangible losses can be difficult to calculate or compensate.

108 REPRODUCTIVE ETHICS IN CLINICAL PRACTICE

23. Paul RG. Damages for wrongful birth and wrongful pregnancy in Illinois. *Loyola Univ Chicago L J.* 1984;15(4):799–842.
24. Ostrom CM. $50m awarded over birth defect: Test said baby would be ok. *The Seattle Times.* 2013 Dec 11.
25. *Grossbaum v. Genesis Genetics Inst., LLC*, 2011 WL 2462279 (D.N.J. 2011).
26. Joel Feinberg has argued that, in certain "extreme cases,"—generally, when the resulting life of the child "is not worth living"—"it is rational to prefer not to have to come into existence at all." Feinberg J. Wrongful conception and the right not be harmed. *Harv J L & Pub Pol'y.* 1985;8:57–77.
27. Costello KR. The limitations of wrongful life claims and genetic diagnosis. *LA Law.* 2007;30:14–18 (only the Supreme Courts of California, Washington, and New Jersey have recognized wrongful life causes of action).
28. See Botkin JR. The legal concept of wrongful life. *JAMA.* 1988;259(10):1541–45.
29. In other words, it may seem easier to bring a wrongful life claim in situations where the embryo has not yet been implanted because one need not focus on balancing fetal interests with the woman's bodily integrity. See Vacco. Preimplantation genetic diagnosis.
30. *Doolan v. IVF America (MA), Inc.*, No. 993476, 2000 WL 33170944 (Mass. Super. Ct. Nov. 20, 2000).
31. Wevers K. Prenatal torts and pre-implantation genetic diagnosis. *Harvard J L & Tech.* 2010;24(1):257–80.
32. *Zepeda v. Zepeda*, 190 N.E.2d 849 (Ill. App. 1963). The court refused to compare the value of existence with the value of nonexistence.
33. What would it mean for abortion law? What would it mean for the law governing the disposition of embryos upon divorce? And even where there is an established duty by the provider to the parents, no court has yet recognized a duty on the part of physicians to inform patients about the option of PGT.
34. *Siemieniec v. Lutheran Gen. Hosp.*, 117 Ill. 2d 230 (Ill. 1987).
35. Adrienne Asch and Erik Parens have famously written that the act of choosing to terminate a pregnancy after prenatal testing reflects the belief "that disability itself, not societal discrimination against people with disabilities, is the problem to be solved." Parens E, Asch A. The disability rights critique of prenatal genetic testing: reflections and recommendations. In Parens E, Asch A., eds., *Prenatal Testing and Disability Rights.* Washington, DC: Georgetown University Press; 2000: 3, 12–13.
36. Wevers. Prenatal torts.
37. In his 1984 book *Reasons and Persons* (Oxford University Press), Derek Parfit presented the hypothetical 14-year-old girl, who chooses to have a baby. He acknowledges that that child will not receive the same start in life had the girl decided to wait several years before having a baby. However, as long as the child is given a life worth living, the child cannot claim to have been harmed by being created.
38. Belsky AJ. Injury as a matter of law: Is this the answer to the wrongful life dilemma? *Univ Baltimore L R.* 1993;22(2):185–268.
39. Hayden EC. Tomorrow's children. *Nature.* 2016;530:402–5. For example, clustered regularly interspaced short palindromic repeats (CRISPR), a technology that

makes it possible to alter the genetic makeup of cells, was named 2015's Science Breakthrough of the Year. See the article: And science's 2015 breakthrough of the year is. *Science.* 2015 Dec 17, http://www.sciencemag.org/news/2015/12/and-science-s-2015-breakthrough-year

40. Cohen IG. Intentional diminishment, the non-identity problem, and legal liability. *Hastings L J.* 2008;60:347.

41. National Academy of Sciences, Engineering, and Medicine. *Human Genome Editing: Science, Ethics, and Governance.* Washington, DC: National Academies Press; 2017. The authors distinguished between preventing disease and "enhancements"— or "changes that go beyond mere restoration or protection of health"—the latter of which it said should not be pursued "at this time."

42. For example, Kirsten Smolensky proposes that wrongful life claims by children against their parents for interfering in their DNA is appropriate when that intervention is "direct" (i.e., where the child is born due to genetic additions, deletions, or modifications that alter the embryo's DNA), but not when the intervention (e.g., PGT) is "indirect." Smolensky KR. Creating children with disabilities: Parental tort liability for preimplantation genetic interventions. *Hastings L J.* 2008;60:299–337. I will leave it to the philosophers to define the line at which a single embryo would become so altered by genetic modification that it would result in a child with a different identity.

7

Who Are Your Patients, and What Happens When They Disagree?

Conflicts in Treating Multiple Parties Engaging in Third-Party Reproduction

Heather E. Ross JD

Jack and Lisa desperately want to have a child. They were referred to your Chicago office 3 years ago and have already been through seven rounds of intrauterine insemination (IUI) and four rounds of in vitro fertilization (IVF). You have recommended they consider working with an egg donor as Lisa is now 41 and was only able to produce three viable eggs during her last retrieval, resulting in one low-quality embryo. The couple considered moving to another fertility clinic in Colorado with higher published pregnancy success rates (you have lost other patients to this clinic) but have decided to remain with you for their last attempt. After this fifth attempt they will deplete their insurance benefits and will need to pay a significant amount out of pocket. You refer them to a local gamete-matching program, and they choose a first-time egg donor from Chicago. The donor visits your office for medical clearance and meets with you briefly. She spends a longer period of time with your staff to discuss the medical protocol. The donor responds well to the stimulation medications and her follicles multiply rapidly, suggesting a successful retrieval with many eggs. She is monitored every other morning by your nursing staff, and you review the results in the afternoon and relay them to Jack and Lisa. The next time you see the donor is for the retrieval. She produces 19 viable eggs resulting in 15 embryos. Jack and Lisa are thrilled because this provides them with plenty of embryos to hopefully achieve a successful pregnancy. The morning after the retrieval, the donor calls your office to complain of severe bloating and nausea. The nurse advises her to come to the office the next day unless she starts feeling worse, in which case she should go to the nearest emergency room. A few hours later you receive a call from an ER physician advising you that the donor has presented bloated and nauseous. She is given an IV, undergoes paracentesis (removing fluid from the belly), and is released from the ER several hours later. You receive a report the following morning from the ER that the donor has been released and is back at home. You do not hear from the donor again.

After five embryo transfer attempts Lisa is unable to maintain a successful pregnancy. You suggest they consider gestational surrogacy. Lisa's friend, Suzy, offers to carry their child for no compensation. You are aware that Suzy is opposed to terminating or reducing a pregnancy for any reason except to save her life. Jack and Lisa have five embryos left, all of which have been PGS tested and appear to be free of genetic abnormalities. The parties agree to transfer two embryos. The transfer is successful, and, at the third ultrasound, you discover one of the embryos has split, resulting in a triplet pregnancy. Suzy's obstetrician believes Suzy will not be able to carry a triplet pregnancy to term and recommends reducing to protect Suzy's health and to increase the chances of a viable pregnancy. Although the parties agreed by contract that they would not terminate or reduce for any reason, Jack and Lisa had not considered the possibility of a triplet pregnancy and do not like the idea of Suzy carrying triplets, especially if it means losing the pregnancy or an early delivery with resulting complications to the babies. Lisa comes to you requesting a reduction, but Suzy is vehemently opposed. Fortunately for you, the identical twin pregnancy is lost at week 11, and Suzy ends up with a singleton pregnancy that proceeds without any medical complications until week 35, when Suzy experiences terrible cramping and starts bleeding. She is rushed to the hospital and the physician on call recommends an immediate caesarean section as the baby's heart rate is dropping. Suzy does not believe in medical intervention and advises the doctor she will not agree to a caesarean. Jack and Lisa are shocked and tell the physician that they must perform the caesarean to save their baby's life.

Does the short amount of time the physician spent with the donor suggest that her health risks may have been minimized, especially in light of her later complication? Does the long term relationship between the physician and Jack and Lisa create a conflict of interest for the physician to also treat the donor? Should Suzy have been required to reduce the triplet pregnancy if it had proceeded? Should Suzy be required to have a caesarean? What rights, if any, do Jack and Lisa have to protect the health of this fetus?

Physician Conflicts of Interest in Egg Donation Arrangements

Although Jack and Lisa and their nonidentified egg donor have a unified purpose—obtaining viable embryos that will result in a successful pregnancy and birth—the means to achieve this outcome has inherent conflicts. The primary goal of Jack and Lisa is to create as many embryos as possible in one cycle so they can create multiple chances at achieving pregnancy in the most cost-effective way possible. The primary goal of the second patient, the egg donor, is to preserve her own health while also completing her donation. Many intended parent(s) can only afford one cycle of egg donation and, like Jack and Lisa, have experienced tremendous psychological and financial hardship and loss even before the use of donor eggs is recommended. In most practices, the physician treats both the intended parent(s) and the egg donor, and typically the physician has known and treated the intended parent(s) through their hardship and loss long before the egg donor becomes a patient. Moreover, the donor's contractual and financial relationship with the intended parent(s) may cause (consciously or unconsciously) the physician to view the donor as a contractor rather than a patient—a mistaken view of the physician's role.

In addition, the laws—or lack thereof—may fuel this conflict. Federal law requires each fertility clinic to report success rates in order to "help infertility patients make informed decisions about assisted reproductive technology"[1]. This federal mandate creates a financial incentive for clinics to achieve positive fertility outcomes and birth rates (i.e., the higher the rate the better advertising of the clinic which is why Jack and Lisa considered switching to the Colorado clinic because of that clinic's higher success rates).[2] There is no corollary requirement to report any statistics on the medical affects or outcomes for egg donors such as medical complications, amount of drugs used, number of eggs retrieved, hyperstimulation, informed consent, etc. Suzy's complications are not reported anywhere. The reporting of these statistics might give potential donors reasons to go to, or avoid, particular doctors or clinics and also the treating physicians to learn from these outcomes and determine whether they are preventable. In fact, the only other existing federal regulations deal solely with safety testing to protect intended parent(s) from donor transmission of communicable diseases to recipients. Although a few states have protective legislation (see later discussion), and the American Society for Reproductive Medicine (ASRM), a self-regulating association, has recommendations for informed consent in egg donor cycles, there are no federal laws and few state laws that regulate informed consent or what information must be provided to women who wish to donate their eggs and no mandated follow-up reporting to study the long-term effects of egg donation.[3]

In short, legal requirements and business imperatives increase the possibility that the medical needs of the egg donor may be consciously or unconsciously minimized in order to maximize the chances of a successful pregnancy.

How should a physician address this potential conflict, and what safeguards can be put in place to ensure the best care possible to both intended parent(s) and egg donor patients? Two areas that offer guidance include living organ donation and the parameters set by the legal community for third-party reproductive arrangements.

Organ donation may be the most analogous medical situation to gamete donation (despite the difference of ability to receive compensation in gamete donation). The Organ Procurement and Transplantation Network (OPTN) was created in 1984 by the National Organ Transplant Act (NOTA) to increase the number of and access to transplants, improve survival rates after transplantation, and promote living donor and transplant recipient safety and efficient management of the system.

OPTN requires an independent living donor advocate (ILDA) to ensure living organ donors are fully informed of the health risks.[4] Specifically, for any living donor who is undergoing evaluation for donation, the living donor recovery hospital must designate and provide each living donor with an ILDA who is not involved with the potential recipient evaluation and is independent of the decision to transplant the potential recipient. There are specific training and qualification requirements for the ILDA concerning knowledge about hospital protocol, medical ethics, informed consent, and the impact of external pressure on the donor's decision to donate. The ILDA must also document and confirm that the donor has received information about the informed consent process, evaluation process, surgical procedures, and will abide by follow-up requirements.

In short, the field of living organ donation imposes several safeguards to prevent the physician's emotional investment in the recipient patient's survival and their reputational and financial stake in their transplant center's success rates from improperly influencing their assessment and recommendations to the living donor, thus avoiding a conflict of interest that could impact the living donor's medical care or decision to donate.

Concerns regarding the conflict of interest that arises when one professional is responsible for the best interest of two parties with potentially conflicting interests in a transaction have also been addressed in the legal field. Both the ethics rules of the American Bar Association (ABA) and the Academy of Adoption and Assisted Reproduction Attorneys (AAAA) prohibit attorneys from representing more than one client in a matter if there is an actual conflict of interest between the parties. AAAA's ethics code states that "In every ART Matter in which a Fellow represents a Party, the other Party(ies) must also have independent legal counsel except: (2) A Fellow may represent (i) both Intended Parents, (ii) a Donor and Donor's spouse or partner or (iii) a Surrogate and Surrogate's spouse or partner *provided that there is no actual conflict of interest* and the potential conflict of interest has been disclosed and waived."[5] Rule 1.7 of the ABA Model Rules of Professional Responsibility provides that "a lawyer shall not represent a client if the representation involves a concurrent conflict of interest." A concurrent conflict of interest exists if the representation of one client will be directly adverse to another client or there is a *significant risk* that the representation of one or more clients will be materially limited by the lawyer's responsibilities to another client. An exception does exist if the lawyer reasonably believes that they will be able to provide competent and diligent representation to each affected client, *and* each affected client gives informed consent, confirmed in writing.

Certain state laws also mandate safeguards for women who wish to donate their eggs. The Illinois Parentage Act requires that egg donors and intended parent(s) have separate and independent legal representation and that a legal agreement be entered into before any embryos are transferred to the recipient.[6] Arizona requires the physician to provide egg donor patients with a detailed description of the medications, hormones, procedures, and potential risks, and advise of the existence of unknown risks, prior to any testing or treatment. Failure to comply with the law may result in actionable consequences, including license suspension or revocation."[7] New York law also codified the necessity for egg donor informed consent prior to a donation, requiring written informed consent "after the director or a designee has provided information to the donor on the procedures for collection, storage and use of semen, oocytes or embryos, and the risks of any drugs, surgical procedures and/or anesthesia administered."[8] California passed legislation in 2010 requiring all persons or entities advertising for paid egg donors to include notification that

Not all potential egg donors are selected. Not all selected egg donors receive the monetary amounts or compensation advertised. As with any medical procedure, there may be risks associated with human egg donation. Before an egg donor agrees to begin the egg donation process, and signs a legally binding contract, she is required to receive specific information on the known risks of egg donation. Consultation with your doctor prior to entering into a donor contract is advised.[9]

Egg donors would be better served if the medical community mirrored protections afforded to living organ donors and followed the rules imposed by lawyers in the field of third-party reproduction to ensure egg donors receive independent, quality medical care. Larger fertility clinics with several physicians on staff could do this by assigning the egg donor to a different physician than the intended parent(s). Another step would be to train an employee of the fertility clinic who is not directly associated with the treating physicians, or an outside expert, to provide independent advice and guidance to the egg donor throughout the process. This individual or team should confirm that the donor is aware of the potential conflicts inherent in egg donation arrangements and is fully informed about both the known and unknown medical and mental health risks associated with egg donation.

Gestational Surrogacy Arrangements

This case study is filled with ethical minefields for which no definitive legal answers exist, and any decisions made will likely result in emotional distress to one or more of the participants and/or physical harm to this fetus. For these reasons, prevention is the best tool available. The risk of conflict can be reduced by requiring the parties to meet with independent attorneys and mental health professionals prior to any medical treatment. Intended parent(s) and the gestational surrogate (and her spouse or partner when applicable) should meet independently and as a group with a mental health professional who has expertise in gestational surrogacy to discuss all aspects and "what if" scenarios of how the arrangement will proceed. Assuming the parties are cleared and found to be appropriate candidates and a good match, they should then meet with independent lawyers to memorialize in writing their specific agreements with respect to medical treatment and all other issues that may arise. The surrogacy agreement should include specific language with respect to how many embryos will be transferred and whether or not the gestational surrogate will submit to various medical procedures (i.e., ultrasound, amniocentesis, cesarean section, termination, selective reduction, etc.). Most agreements provide that if the gestational surrogate's life or health is not in danger, she will submit to procedures requested by the intended parent(s) that are medically indicated to protect the pregnancy and fetus but that, ultimately, her health and safety will take precedence over that of the gestated fetus. The most challenging task for lawyers drafting and reviewing surrogacy agreements is to preserve the gestational surrogate's right to bodily autonomy while addressing the intended parent's desire to make medical decisions concerning the fetus. A carefully drafted agreement will guide the parties on how medical decisions will be made and what will happen if the parties do not agree. In most cases, engaging in the process of articulating each party's desires and expectations, negotiating compromises, putting them in writing, and signing avoids future disagreement between the parties. Nonetheless, situations may arise not contemplated by any of the parties (or attorneys), and/or participants may change their minds once confronted with a medical decision.

There are two potential sources of law in this area: statutes passed by legislatures, and opinions written by judges ("case law"). Although no case law exists with respect to medical issues in the context of a gestational surrogacy arrangement, there are cases that address a pregnant woman's right to bodily autonomy and cases that address a parent's right to protect their child. How these separate areas of case law might interact in a surrogacy conflict is an open question. It is important to note that the field of gestational surrogacy is vastly different from that of adoption, and this chapter does not address adoption. In adoption, a woman carrying a genetically-related child she typically created by accident decides she cannot parent that child. In contrast, a child born by gestational surrogacy would not exist but for two intentional acts—the intended parent(s) creation of embryos genetically related to them (and not related to the gestational surrogate), and the gestational surrogate's choice to attempt to gestate the embryo(s) for the sole purpose of enabling the intended parent(s) to parent the resulting child. Therefore, adoption law is not usually considered relevant to the analysis of conflicts between intended parents and gestational surrogates.

The US Supreme Court has held that a person has a constitutionally protected right to refuse unwanted medical treatment or procedures and, in one instance, has refused to give a genetic stakeholder, the husband, the power to interfere in the abortion decision.[10] In *Planned Parenthood of Southeastern Pennsylvania v. Casey*,[11] the Court found that a husband's notification could not be required in order for his wife to obtain an abortion, noting, "if the husband's interest in the fetus' safety is a sufficient predicate for state regulation, the State could reasonably conclude that pregnant wives should notify their husbands before drinking alcohol or smoking."[12] Because the Court struck down a state's attempt to allow a pregnant woman's spouse to have a voice in her medical decisions, it may be unlikely that such regulation would be extended to intended parent(s) in a gestational surrogacy arrangement, despite their genetic connection to the fetus.

However, the Supreme Court has also held that parents have a constitutionally protected fundamental liberty interest in procreation and "the care, custody and management of their child."[13] What the US Supreme Court has not considered is whether this interest extends to decision-making for a fetus gestated in a non-parent's body.

The *Casey* decision was premised partly on the notion of a woman's right to liberty guaranteed by the Constitution, including her right to decide her own destiny about whether or not she will create a child.

> The mother who carries a child to full term is subject to anxieties, to physical constraints, to pain that only she must bear. That these sacrifices have from the beginning of the human race been endured by woman with a pride that ennobles her in the eyes of others and gives to the infant a bond of love cannot alone be grounds for the State to insist she make the sacrifice. Her suffering is too intimate and personal for the State to insist, without more, upon its own vision of the woman's role, however dominant that vision has been in the course of our history and our culture. The destiny of the woman must be shaped to a large extent on her own conception of her spiritual imperatives and her place in society.

If the rationale supporting this right to "liberty" is nonexistent for a gestational surrogate (as she will not be the parent to the resulting child) it is possible a court will not follow *Casey* if faced with a pregnant surrogate refusing medical treatment.

Roe v. Wade[14] is the landmark decision granting a pregnant woman, along with her physician, the right to make decisions with respect to her pregnancy, including the right to terminate prior to fetal viability. *Roe* recognized, however, that a state could have a compelling interest in the potential life of a fetus after viability ("if the State is interested in protecting fetal life after viability, it may go so far as to proscribe abortion during that period, except when it is necessary to preserve the life or health of the mother").[15] Since a state has the authority to proscribe post-viability abortion, would some courts be willing to require medical intervention to protect the health of the fetus at the request of the genetic and intended parents, as opposed to the request of a doctor? The answer to this question may depend on the type of medical treatment requested or refused and the state in which the pregnant woman resides.

Court decisions differ from state to state with respect to whether a state's interest in protecting fetal life can override a women's right to bodily autonomy. For example, upholding a women's right to refuse a cesarean delivery at 35 weeks' gestation despite the physician's recommendation that the fetus was not receiving adequate oxygen, an Illinois appellate court held that "a woman is under no duty to guarantee the mental and physical health of her child at birth, and thus cannot be compelled to do or not do anything merely for the benefit of her unborn child."[16] In this 1994 Illinois opinion, the court suggested that if the medical treatment had not been as invasive (i.e., had it been a blood transfusion), it may have decided differently. However, 3 years later, another Illinois appellate court extended the cesarean rationale to all medical procedures, finding that "a blood transfusion is an invasive medical procedure that interrupts a competent adult's bodily integrity" and that Illinois courts cannot not override a competent woman's decisions regarding any medical treatment to potentially save the life of a viable fetus.[17]

None of these cases contemplated surrogacy, and in all previous cases the woman refusing the cesarean delivery or the blood transfusion, or requesting the abortion, was making a medical decision affecting the health of her own child and her own right to parent. Perhaps the court would have reached a different conclusion if the gestated fetus would eventually be the legal child of a third party and the gestational surrogate had contractually agreed to undergo the medical procedure. Or, perhaps this fact will make no difference at all, as a 1990 opinion from the DC court, finding that a woman cannot be ordered to have a caesarean section to protect the life of her fetus, based its decision partly on the concern that court-ordered medical treatments "erode the element of trust that permits a pregnant woman to communicate with her physician without fear of reprisal."[18] Court-ordered intervention may result in a woman who has complications or is at high risk to avoid communicating honestly with her doctor for fear that she will be ordered to engage in unwanted medical treatment.

Although the majority of jurisdictions have followed the same reasoning as the Illinois court, protecting a pregnant woman's right to bodily autonomy,[19] it is not universal. For example, in *Jefferson v. Griffin Spalding County Hospital Authority*, the Georgia Supreme Court authorized the hospital plaintiff to perform a cesarean delivery where the mother's refusal at 39 weeks' gestation based on religious grounds was predicted to cause almost certain fetal death.[20] And, in *Crouse Irving Memorial Hospital, Inc. v. Paddock*, a New York court ordered blood transfusions over religious objection to save the mother and fetus.[21] Therefore, a Georgia or New York court may be more willing to order Suzy to comply with medical procedures agreed to by contract and in the best medical interest of the fetus than a court sitting in Illinois, Washington DC, or Massachusetts.

A few states address the issue of bodily autonomy by statute. For example, the surrogacy statute in Illinois provides that the gestational surrogate has the right to choose her physician (after consultation with the intended parent[s]), but does not specifically state that a gestational surrogate maintains bodily autonomy. In fact, the Illinois statute allows the parties to include contractual provisions that a gestational surrogate agree to fetal monitoring, testing, and treatment recommended by her physician. It is possible that this could be interpreted to mean that an Illinois gestational surrogate is permitted to contract away her right to bodily autonomy.[22]However, the recent passage of the Illinois Reproductive Health Act ("IL-RHA"), which became law 15 years after the Illinois surrogacy statute, may impact the enforcement of the contractual rights of parties to a surrogacy agreement because the IL-RHA provides pregnant individuals full autonomy to make decisions about reproductive health and restricts the ability of the State to interfere with these fundamental rights.[23]

Other state statutes have explicitly addressed the gestational surrogate's right to make medical decisions. The Texas surrogacy statute states "a gestational agreement may not limit the right of the gestational mother to make decisions to safeguard her health or the health of an embryo."[24] The Florida statute attempts to provide protection for both the gestational surrogate's bodily autonomy and the fetus, stating that "the commissioning couple agrees that the gestational surrogate shall be the sole source of consent with respect to clinical intervention and management of the pregnancy" *and* that "the gestational surrogate agrees to submit to reasonable medical evaluation and treatment and to adhere to reasonable medical instructions about her prenatal health."[25] Notably, New York recently passed a surrogacy law that includes a surrogate's bill of rights, which has been quoted as having the "strongest protections for surrogates in the nation." Accordingly, prior New York cases ordering a pregnant person to comply with physician ordered medical treatment may be decided differently today, and would likely not be extended to a gestational surrogate.[26]

In addition to the open constitutional questions, the possibility of enforcing a court order for treatment is horrifying to most. (Would the police go to the home of a surrogate who resisted a court order to abort or to have a Cesarean section and arrest her? Would doctors physically restrain a screaming woman and do the procedure against her will? Thankfully, both are hard to picture.) Therefore, perhaps the issue is not whether a gestational surrogate may contract away her right to make decisions affecting her bodily autonomy (because this should never be allowed) but whether she may contract away her right to receive compensation or expense reimbursement if she refuses to abide by previously agreed-to terms concerning the health of the fetus. If a gestational surrogate who agreed to a physician recommended cesarean section refuses, would a court allow compensation or expense reimbursement to be cut off? Would a lawsuit brought by intended parent(s) for damages to the child be upheld if the child is born with complications directly related to the refusal to have a cesarean section?

Because courts have not addressed the issue of bodily autonomy in the context of a surrogacy arrangement, requiring patients to meet with separate lawyers and to memorialize their intent with respect to medical procedures in a written document and have mental health consultations may well be the most important steps a physician can take to avoid future conflict. In the event a conflict does arise, consulting a legal expert and seeking guidance from a court prior to medical treatment is the best course of action.

References

1. See https://www.fertilityauthority.com/articles/fertility-clinic-success-rates
2. Bass C, Gregorio J. Conflicts of interest for physicians treating egg donors. *AMA J Ethics*. 2014 Oct;16(10):822–6, http://journalofethics.ama-assn.org/2014/10/pfor2-1410.html2; Fertility Clinic Success Rate and Certification Act, 42 USC 263a-1 (1992).

3. American Medical Association. Virtual mentor. *AMA J Ethics*. January 2014 Jan;16(1):49–56, http://journalofethics.ama-assn.org/2014/01/hlaw2-1401.html.
4. The Organ Procurement and Transplantation Network. Guidance for the informed consent of living donors, http://optn.transplant.hrsa.gov/ContentDocuments/.
5. See AAAA Ethics Code, Rule 16 (a)(2).
6. Illinois Gestational Surrogacy Act 750 ILCS 47/et. seq. (2005).
7. Ariz Rev Stat Ann sec 36–1702 (West 2010).
8. Informed consent, NY Comp Codes R & Regs title 10, sec 52–8.8(a) (2000).
9. Oocyte donation; advertisement; screening process; procedures, Cal Health and safety Code sec 125325 (West 2010).
10. *Cruzan v. Director, Mo. Health Department*, 497 US 261 (1990) (Supreme Court stated that this right derives from the Fourteenth Amendment, which provides that no State shall "deprive any person of life, liberty, or property, without due process of law.") See also, *In re Estate of Longeway*, 123 Ill. 2d 33, 549 N.E. 2d 292 (1989) (Supreme Court of Illinois found that a 76-year-old woman rendered incompetent from a series of strokes had a right [by request of her guardian] to the discontinuance of artificial nutrition and hydration, treating artificial nutrition and hydration as medical treatment.)
11. *Planned Parenthood v. Casey,* 505 U.S. 833, 898 (1992).
12. Ibid., 898.
13. *Skinner v. Oklahoma*, 316 U.S. 535 (1942) (striking down legislation allowing for sterilization, the Court found that "marriage and procreation are fundamental to the very existence and survival of the race"). See also, *Santosky v. Kramer*, 455 U.S. 745, 753–4 (1982) (natural parents have a fundamental liberty interest in "the care, custody and management of their child"). See also, *Stanley v. Illinois*, 405 U.S. 645, 652 (1972) (the right to conceive and raise one's children is deemed essential and the "basic civil rights of man"), citing *Skinner v. Oklahoma*, 316 U.S. 535 at 541.
14. *Roe v. Wade*, 410 U.S. 113 (1973).
15. Ibid., 163–164.
16. *In re Baby Doe,* 632 N.E.2d 326, 332 (1st Dist. 1994).
17. *In re Fetus Brown* 689 N.E.2d 397, 405 (1st Dist. 1997).
18. *In re A.C.* 573 A.2d 1235 (D.C. Court of Appeals 1990).
19. *In re Fetus Brown* 689 N.E.2d 397 at 405 ("State may not override a pregnant women's competent treatment decision, including refusal of recommended invasive medical procedures, to potentially save the life of a viable fetus"). See also, *In re A.C.* 573 A.2d 1235 (rights of the fetus should not be balanced against the rights of the mother); *Taft v. Taft* 446 N.E.2d 395 (Mass.1983) (it is a violation of a pregnant woman's constitutional right to privacy to order her to have her cervix stitched to prevent a miscarriage).
20. *Jefferson v. Griffin Spalding County Hospital Authority* 274 S.E.2d 457 (Ga. 1981).
21. *Crouse Irving Memorial Hospital, Inc. v. Paddock*, 485 N.Y.S.2d 443 (1985) (blood transfusions ordered over religious objection to save the mother and fetus).

22. Ross HE. Gestational surrogacy in Illinois: Contracting the unknown. J DuPage County Bar. 2013–2014;26,16–22. http://www.dcba.org/mpage/vol261213art1.
23. Illinois Reproductive Health Act, 775 ILCS 55/1-15.
24. Texas Family Code Annotated 160.754(f).
25. 2011 Florida Statute 742.15(2) (a) and (b).
26. Chuck E. New York state, long a holdout against legalizing surrogacy, overturns ban. NBC News. April 3, 2020, https://www.nbcnews.com/news/us-news/new-york-state-long-holdout-against-legalizing-surrogacy-overturns-ban-n1176071

8

Ethical Issues in Oocyte Donation

Susan C. Klock PhD

In 1983, for the first time in the evolution of the human species, a woman could give birth to a child that was not created from her own oocyte.[1] In this case the donor underwent superovulation and had her eggs retrieved and inseminated with the intended father's sperm to create embryos. The embryos were transferred into the intended mothers' uterus and a pregnancy resulted. This profound milestone has created a new area of assisted reproductive technology. Oocyte donation allowed for the reproductive process to be broken down into its component parts (genetic mother, gestating mother, and rearing mother) and introduced the inclusion of a third party for female infertility.

In addition to these new reproductive roles, oocyte donation has prompted several ethical concerns which are the focus of this chapter. A brief review of infertility and the clinical process of oocyte donation is presented, then three ethical controversies are discussed: (1) payment to oocyte donors, (2) donors' post-donation medical and psychological well-being, and (3) privacy and disclosure to gamete-donation children.

Introduction

In a review of international population surveys, Boivin et al. estimated that 3.5–16.7% of women of childbearing age have some form of infertility.[2] In addition to the base rate of infertility, there has been a trend over the past 3 decades for women to delay childbearing.[3] This trend, combined with the decline of female fertility after the age of 35 has led to the expansion of reproductive technologies. The era of assisted reproduction began in 1978, with the birth of Louise Brown after in vitro fertilization (IVF), followed quickly in 1983 with the first oocyte donor pregnancy.[1] According to the most recent Centers for Disease Control (CDC) and Society of Assisted Reproductive

Technology (SART) data, in 2018, of 306,197 total IVF cycles, 2368 (<1%) were with fresh embryos created from fresh donated eggs, 3362 (1%) were with embryos created from previously frozen eggs, and 14,226 (4.6%) used thawed embryos created with donated eggs.[4]

Oocyte donation is used for women with advanced maternal age, decreased ovarian reserve, and heritable genetic disorders as well as for men in same-sex couples. Oocyte donation has provided the opportunity of parenthood through pregnancy to individuals previously unable to reach this goal. The American Society for Reproductive Medicine (ASRM) has published practice guidelines for oocyte donation since 1998. The most re-cent version provides clinical recommendations for the screening and selec-tion of both oocyte donors and recipients.[5] Briefly, oocyte donors are women between 21 and 34 years of age, with proven fertility desired but not required, who have completed a medical and psychological screening process. The medical screening includes a complete personal and health history, a phys-ical exam, and laboratory testing. The psychological screening includes a clinical interview and psychological testing.[5] Donor psychological exclusion criteria include major psychiatric illness, family history of heritable psychi-atric disorder, substance abuse or dependence, current use of psychoactive medications, history of sexual or physical abuse without treatment, impaired cognitive functioning, and inability to give informed consent.

In contrast to the increasing numbers of potential recipients, it can be dif-ficult to recruit and maintain suitable donors. German et al. found that of 1,114 telephone inquiries from women interested in donating their oocytes, 24% of 364 women who completed background questionnaires were interviewed, 36 stayed in the program, and 14 (1.3%) completed a donation cycle.[6] These rates of attrition through the screening process are typical. Due to the resource-intensive nature of the screening process, programs are inter-ested in donor retention. The ASRM Practice Committee guidelines indicate that donors can donate up to six times,[7] but one study has indicated that most donors donate one or two times.[8]

The clinical process for intended parents is lengthy and requires medical and psychological consultation as well.[5] After the couple selects a donor and the match is made, legal contracts are created delineating financial issues; rights and responsibilities for the eggs and resulting embryos, including disposition of unused embryos; and information-sharing between the in-tended parents, the donor, and the future child. From the time of the ini-tial inquiry about oocyte donation to the completion of the screening for all parties, matching, and legal consultation, the process can take between 3 and 9 months. This often comes after years of infertility treatment, and therefore intended parents can pressure agencies and programs to have many donors available for their immediate use, leading to increased "supply and demand" pressure.

Ethical Issues

Is Paid Donation Voluntary?

The first case of oocyte donation in 1983 was a sister-to-sister donation.[1] During the 1980s and early 1990s, known donors or women undergoing tubal ligation were frequent sources of donated oocytes, and compensation was not provided. Demand soon outstripped supply, and IVF programs and egg donor agencies began recruiting and compensating donors.[9] The legal backdrop for the compensation of oocyte donors is the 1984 National Organ Transplant Act,[10] which banned payment for human organs or tissue but allowed "reasonable payments associated with the removal, transportation, implantation, processing" of the tissue. Initial amounts of about $250 were reported as egg donation emerged as a new treatment option, but compensation quickly rose.[11] Some countries banned egg donation entirely (Germany, Norway, Sweden, and Japan), other countries allowed egg donation but banned payment to donors (Canada, United Kingdom, France, and some Australian states), while the United States, Turkey, the Czech Republic, and South Africa, among others, allow compensation to donors.

In 2007, the average donor compensation was $4,200.[12] Concerns in the field emerged regarding higher compensation given to donors with preferred qualities, "proven donors," or repeat donors. Additionally, in the absence of any regulations governing donor recruitment and compensation, individuals or couples seeking specific characteristics were commonly found online with promises of exorbitant ($25,000–50,000) compensation. These high compensation amounts highlighted the fact that most donors were students or were from the lower income range while the recipients tended to be from higher income levels. High compensation amounts were hotly debated, and concerns about financial coercion of donors emerged.[13,14]

In 2007, the Ethics Committee of the ASRM issued a statement presenting their opinion about compensation to donors, stating that it was justified but should be structured to reflect the time, effort, and discomfort that a donor undergoes.[11] This document also indicated that compensation of more than $5,000 required justification and that more than $10,000 was not appropriate.

In 2014, donors organized and brought a class action law suit against the ASRM for price fixing and unfair competitive practices, targeting their compensation guidelines. In 2016, the ASRM agreed to a settlement and removed language from their guidelines setting compensation levels.[15] The 2016 guidelines call for programs to continue to structure compensation to reflect the time and burden a donor undergoes and not link compensation to the number of eggs, characteristics of the donor, or the outcome of previous cycles. Despite these recommendations, the compensation of donors continues to climb. Donor compensation varies, but amounts of $7,000–8,500 are typical for first-time donors.

Is it ethical to compensate donors for their oocytes? Arguments for the payment of donors include that it is fair to donors to compensate them for their time, effort, and discomfort. Sperm donors have been compensated for decades, between $50 and $100 per sample for a donation process that involves much less time and effort than oocyte donation. Undergoing a donation cycle is difficult, requiring injectable medications, frequent visits to the fertility clinic for ultrasounds and blood tests, and undergoing a minimally invasive surgical procedure to collect the eggs; therefore, many believe payment consistent with currents levels is appropriate to provide egg donors similar benefit to sperm donors. Those in favor of payment argue that most women would not undergo these procedures without compensation, and, in countries without donor compensation, the waiting lists are long and there is an active practice of "reproductive tourism" in which couples travel to countries that have a greater supply of (compensated) donors. The demand for oocytes typically exceeds the supply, thus driving compensation levels higher. Therefore, another argument for payment is to attract new donors or retain repeat donors (thus decreasing recruitment and screening costs). Donors and programs may also perceive that a premium can be paid to donors with proven fertility. Additionally, donors are knowledgeable about the removal of compensation limits and are free to set their own compensation levels.

Arguments against any payment of donors posit that it is a commodification of life and that unique individual reproductive tissue cannot have a price placed upon it. Additionally, payment may undermine the feelings of altruism that prompt the donor to donate, thus creating cognitive dissonance between her altruistic motive and the receipt of monetary compensation.

Last, payment to donors makes egg donation a treatment that is only available to those with the economic resources; thus expense continues to be a barrier to treatment for others from less advantageous economic backgrounds.

In considering whether payment to donors is coercive we must consider the autonomy of women to make decisions about their own bodies. If, after thorough counseling, a woman decides to be a donor, then she should have the option to do that. The concern regarding coercion increases as compensation goes up: a donor may decide that $5,000 is not enough money for her to consider the risks of donation, but for $10,000 or more, she may decide to proceed. This could prompt donors to make decisions that are not beneficial to their well-being. That is why the removal of the compensation cap in 2016 represents what could be the beginning of the slippery slope of coercive compensation. Last, from a justice perspective, oocyte donation is a scare resource and is not equally distributed to all individuals who may want it or benefit from it. It is a treatment for people with resources.

Is Oocyte Donation Safe?

Since the establishment of oocyte donation, clinicians and researchers have been concerned about the donors' post-donation physical and mental well-being. Interest in the well-being of egg donors is a significant concern because the donor—a young, healthy woman—undergoes a medical procedure for which she does not receive any health benefit; therefore, establishing that she does not suffer any harm is of great importance. This section will review what is known about the physical and emotional risks of egg donation for the donor.

The most comprehensive review of the risks of egg donation was completed in 2006, when the Institute of Medicine (IOM) convened a panel, of which this author was a member, reviewing the risks of egg donation in the context of oocyte donation for research and concluded oocyte donation is relatively safe from a physical perspective.[16] And while oocyte donation for research is different from that for clinical purposes, the medical risks are the same. The IOM report identified three short-term medical risks: ovarian hyperstimulation syndrome (OHSS), surgical risks such as bleeding or infection related to the egg retrieval procedure, and risks related to sedation. OHSS refers to a condition in which the ovaries hyperstimulate and enlarge, with the woman experiencing bloating, discomfort, nausea, and/or diarrhea.

It can be classified as mild, moderate, severe, or critical. Cases that are severe or critical can require hospitalization and lead to serious illness and, in rare cases, death. The risk of OHSS is estimated to occur in approximately 1–2% of cases.[6] Maxwell et al.[17] found mild OHSS in 5.9% of a sample of 886 donor retrieval cycles, whereas Soderstrom-Anttila[18] reported it to be 5% in 582 donations. A recent report has described how to identify and minimize risks of OHSS.[19] Other risks associated with oocyte retrieval include bleeding, infection, or ovarian torsion and are estimated as occurring in less than 0.5% of cases.[16] Anesthesia risks are related to the use of sedation for the egg retrieval procedure and are rare.[16]

The long-term medical risks are more difficult to quantify but are thought to include compromised ovarian reserve or infertility and the possibility of cancer. It has been reported that 11.5% of donors were unsuccessful in conceiving naturally 1 year after their donation, and 5% of past donors have sought infertility treatment themselves.[18] Kramer et al. reported that 9% of their sample of 155 donors reported post-donation infertility,[20] thus suggesting that donation does not affect future fertility. No study to date has accurately quantified whether oocyte donation affects future fertility.

Another possible long-term medical risk to donors is cancer. The IOM report concluded that an increased risk of cancer is a "plausible" concern, but it is unknown whether young women exposed to fertility medications in the context of egg donation would have a greater cancer risk. There have been two case reports of the occurrence of gastrointestinal cancer after donation.[21,22] In both these reported cases, the donor developed gastrointestinal cancer four years after donation. Long-term follow-up studies are needed to determine if there are in fact increased long-term health risks to donors.

In addition to donors' post-donation physical well-being, limited retrospective studies have investigated donors' psychological adjustment. The short-term psychological concerns are mood swings that frequently accompany the ovulation stimulation medications, anxiety related to medication injections, preprocedure retrieval anxiety, and emotional reactions to interactions with clinic staff. Soderstrom-Anttila reported that 3.3% of their sample of 428 donors reported transient mood symptoms during the donation cycle, but, overall, almost all donors (99%) were satisfied or very satisfied with their decision to donate, and 95% would recommend it to other women.[18] Kenney and McGowan reported that 15% of their sample of 80 donors reported mood changes during their donation cycle.[23] Long-term psychological risks include regret about donating, anxiety about not knowing the outcome of the donation, or fear of having future contact with the child. Kenney and McGowan also reported that 20% of their 80 donors reported having lasting psychological effects from the donation, including curiosity about the outcome and concerns that the child from their donation cycle might develop a relationship with the donor's child. On a positive note, three donors reported ongoing pride that they had helped an infertile couple have a child.[23] Jordan et al. reported that, among their sample of 24 previous donors, 17% had an "intense" desire to know whether a pregnancy resulted from their donation, and 37% had concerns about the parenting style of the recipients.[24]

The ethical implications of donor well-being are concerning on several levels. First, in the interest of beneficence and nonmaleficence, the field of assisted reproduction should focus its attention and resources to further understand the long-term impact of oocyte donation on donors' health. The commercial interest to recruit and use donors should be counterbalanced by research on donor well-being. Large, prospective studies could provide information to donors and providers to assure the safety of the procedure or identify previously unknown risks. Additionally, in the interest of patient autonomy, further research is needed to more fully counsel prospective donors on the long-term impacts of donation to allow them to weigh the risks and benefits and aid in their decision-making about whether the compensation is worth the possible risks. When counseling donors, clinicians should go through, in detail, the steps in the donation process and discuss some of the long-term implications, such as: What if a child wants contact in the future? What if they regret the decision? What if a child is conceived by the donation to another couple and in the future the donor is unable to have a child of her own? Donors should have the information and time to consider the medical and psychological risks and benefits of donation if they are to provide informed consent.

How Do You Balance the Needs of Stakeholders?: Information-Sharing, Privacy, and Disclosure

A third area of ethical concern in gamete donation is the issue of privacy or disclosure to offspring regarding their donor gamete origin. A tradition of maintaining privacy regarding gamete donation began with the first clinical case report of sperm donation in the late 1800s and continued until the mid

1980s. The tradition of privacy was supported by physicians and recipients for several reasons. Privacy in gamete donation was grounded in the privacy model traditionally used in adoption. In addition, privacy about gamete donation protected the infertile individual from public awareness of their infertility. Also, privacy prevented the donor from having responsibilities toward the donor child. Last, privacy was thought to maintain a family's sense of cohesion and the feeling that the child "belonged" to them.

In the past, the recommendation to maintain privacy was based on the "best interest of the child" belief. Now, 30 years later, guided by that same principle, there has been a movement toward disclosure about gamete donation. This movement was prompted by several factors. The first was the change in the adoption model, which moved from a closed model to an open model in respect for children's rights to know their biological origin. Second, the increasing use of donor gametes by single women and gay and lesbian couples has necessitated disclosure to the child as the child becomes aware of the facts of reproduction. Third, in 2013, the Ethics Committee of the ASRM explicitly recommended disclosure in donor gamete families.[25] Fourth, the presence of the internet and ready access to information has made maintaining privacy more difficult. Last, legislation in Denmark and the United Kingdom mandating donor registries and disclosure of donor information to the child upon the child reaching the age of 18 has affected the move toward disclosure. All of these changes have been focused on enhancing the well-being of the child.

Despite these efforts toward disclosure there is still variability in what parents actually do in terms of informing their children of their gamete donation origin. As a review in 2016 by Talladini et al. indicated, among egg donor parents 23% having told their child, 48% are planning to tell, and 16% are planning to not tell.[26] The percentages of disclosure to the child are interesting when compared to the percentages of parents who have told other people. Most (58–86%) donor gamete parents have told others about using a donor to conceive,[27–29] but most (60–86%) regretted telling others.[28] When asked, parents regret telling others because they felt that they had less control over the information and they were worried that the child could find out from someone else.

There are several reasons why parents tell their child. Common themes are that the child has a "right to know," "honesty is the best policy," or "we've told so many other people, we have to tell the child." Particularly with the broad availability of home DNA kits and donor information on the internet, the maintenance of privacy about donor-gamete origin children may be an illusion. Alternatively, there are several reasons that parents do not tell, including, "there is no reason to tell, I am the parent," community/ culture would not accept a donor child, and concerns that their child would be perceived as "different." Parents who don't know if they will tell or think they will not tell describe feeling afraid that if their child finds out it will create a rupture in the family, specifically in the relationship with the nongenetically related parent. Additionally, patients from certain communities and cultures feel they absolutely cannot tell the child for fear that the child will be stigmatized and ostracized from the community.

The argument to disclose to a donor child is based in the belief of the best interest of the child. These discussions usually suggest that there will be better psychological adjustment among donor children who are told versus those who are not. Three small studies have investigated this question and found no differences in child adjustment based on disclosure status.[30-32]

Of significant importance in the disclosure debate are the ethical principles of autonomy and beneficence from the viewpoint of the donor-conceived individual. Donor-conceived individuals have the right to information about their genetic origins, particularly now in the age of genomics and genetic-based medicine and health outcomes. Blyth et al. have noted that most adult donor-conceived individuals are interested in having some information about their donor.[33] This includes information about physical and psychological characteristics, reasons for donating, and the identity of the donor. In her recent review, Zweifel has noted that the emerging literature suggests that donor-conceived individuals "vary in the intensity of their desire to learn more about their donor."[34] It is suggested that the interest may be stronger for older individuals and for those who do not have a social father. Ravelingien et al. noted that many donor-conceived individuals are curious about their donors in terms of physical resemblance or personality characteristics.[35] Additionally, they are interested in what kind of individual the donor was and their reasons for donating. A subset of donor-conceived individuals have sought out the identity of their donor on donor–offspring sites, such as the Donor Sibling Registry, and donor offspring and their donors have had contact or have met. These meetings can be rewarding and provide closure or, in some cases, can lead to sadness and disappointment as the imagined meeting does not meet expectations. Additionally, with the more widespread use of direct-to-consumer DNA testing, the ability for donor-conceived people to connect with their donor is increasing. As Braverman and Schlaff point out, all stakeholders need to understand the limits on privacy due to technological advances that can lead to donor connection in a few keystrokes. The availability of information on platforms such as 23andMe and Ancestry is yet another facet in the argument that disclosure to children is recommended.[36]

From the perspective of the child, few can argue that disclosure is not required. However, from the perspective of the parents and the donor, one could argue that disclosure may not be required. Balancing the rights and responsibilities of all stakeholders can more effectively be managed with pre-treatment counseling regarding the short- and long-term implications of gamete donation. Clinicians and agency personnel can counsel donors prior to donation regarding their preferences for disclosure. Agencies can serve as liaisons between donors and offspring to manage the sharing of information when and if the donor-conceived person is interested in having more information. The clinician should discuss privacy and disclosure with the intended parents before and after pregnancy. Although many clinicians feel an obligation to tell intended parents to disclose, this can truncate a full discussion of the issues. The clinician should maintain neutrality to allow the patient(s) to explore their thoughts about disclosure and the positive and negative aspects of both privacy and disclosure. Exploring the pros and cons of both positions can lead the intended parents to clarify their position and help them develop an initial plan for managing the donor information and selecting a donor with similar preferences for disclosure as their own. Also, discussing specific strategies for disclosure and age-appropriate narratives can help lessen anxiety about disclosure and help individuals feel more confident in the disclosure process. Neutrality is also important because attitudes vary over time. If the clinician imposes their opinion on the patient from the outset, patients may not feel free to express their own opinion nor feel comfortable contacting the clinician in the future if they opted for a choice the clinician did not recommend. This is particularly relevant if and when the parents return in the future with their child or when an event has come up that has prompted a re-examination of the disclosure decision. This can happen when a parent(s) returns for counseling during a time of illness or divorce and they need a neutral place to process their feelings and create a new disclosure plan. Last, clinicians can share the perspective that parents' attitudes and plans may change over time, most importantly because their child will influence their disclosure decision by his or her own curiosity, interest, and personality.

Conclusion

Oocyte donation has led to the creations of tens of thousands of children who are genetically unrelated to one or both of their social parents. For the first time in human evolution, a woman can give birth to a child who is not genetically related to her. The increasing use of oocyte donation prompts significant ethical questions for all parties: donors, intended parents, donor-conceived offspring, and the medical professionals who make these arrangements possible. In the United States, the issue of payment to donors continues to provoke questions about appropriate limits to compensation, financial coercion, and autonomy. Worldwide, the topic of donor well-being, both physical and psychological, has received limited attention but requires further study to determine ways to minimize risk. Finally, information sharing between parents, children, and donors continues to develop and evolve. Fundamental to the disclosure decisions by parents of oocyte-donor children is: What makes a parent? Is it the genetic information shared in reproduction or is it the psychosocial relationship formed in the day-to-day rearing and caring for a child as they grow? The dichotomous "nature versus nurture" view in the setting of gamete donation is unhelpfully simplistic. Donor gamete procreation prompts all of us to develop new paradigms to consider the meaning of parenting.

References

1. Trounson A, Leeton J, Besanko M, Wood C, Conti A. Pregnancy established in an infertile patient after transfer of a donated embryo fertilized in vitro. *BMJ*. 1983;286:835–8.
2. Boivin J, Bunting L, Collins JA, Nygren KG. International estimates of infertility prevalence and treatment-seeking: Potential need and demand for infertility medical care. *Hum Reprod*. 2007;22:1506–12.
3. Speroff L, Fritz MA, eds. *Clinical Gynecologic Endocrinology and Infertility*. 8th ed. Philadelphia, PA: Lippincott Williams & Wilkins; 2011: chap. 1.
4. Retrieved from https://www.cdc.gov/art/artdata/index.html.
5. Practice Committee of the American Society for Reproductive Medicine and the Practice Committee of the Society for Assisted Reproductive Technology. Recommendations for gamete and embryo donation: A committee opinion. *Fertil Steril*. 2013;99:47–62.
6. German E, Mukherjee T, Osborne D, Copperman A. Does increasing ovum donor compensation lead to differences in donor characteristics? *Fertil Steril*. 2001;76:75–9.

7. Practice Committee of the American Society for Reproductive Medicine and Practice Committee of the Society for Assisted Reproductive Technology. Repetitive oocyte donation: A committee opinion. *Fertil Steril.* 2014;102:964–6.

8. Klock SC, Elman Stout J, Davidson M. Psychological characteristics and factors related to willingness to donate again among anonymous oocyte donors. *Fertil Steril.* 2003;79:1312–16.

9. Steinbock B. Payment for egg donation and surrogacy. *Mount Sinai J Med.* 2004;71:255–65.

10. National Organ Transplant Act (NOTA;P.L. 98-507), 1984.

11. Ethics Committee of the American Society of Reproductive Medicine. Financial compensation of oocyte donors: An Ethics committee opinion. *Fertil Steril.* 2007;88:305–9.

12. Covington S, Gibbons W, for the Society for Assisted Reproductive Technology. What is happening to the price of eggs? *Fertil Steril.* 2007;87:1001–4.

13. Bergh P. Indecent proposal: $5000 is not "reasonable compensation" for oocyte donors—a reply. *Fertil Steril.* 1999;71:9–10.

14. Daniels K. To give or sell human gametes: The interplay between pragmatics, policy and ethics. *J Medical Ethics.* 2000;26:206–11.

15. Ethics Committee of the American Society of Reproductive Medicine. Financial compensation of oocyte donors: An Ethics committee opinion. *Fertil Steril.* 2016;106:15–19.

16. Institute of Medicine and national Research Council. *Assessing the Medical Risks of Human Oocyte Donation for Stem Cell Research: Workshop Report.* Washington DC: The National Academies Press; 2007. Retrieved from https://doi.org/10.17226/11832

17. Maxwell K, Cholst I, Rosenwaks Z. The incidence of both serious and minor complications in young women undergoing oocyte donation. *Fertil Steril.* 2008;90:2165–71.

18. Soderstrom-Anttila V, Miettinen A, Rotkirch A, Nuojua-Huttunen S, Paranen A, Salevaara M, Suikkari A. Short and long-term health consequences and current satisfaction levels for altruistic anonymous, identity-release and known oocyte donors. *Human Reprod.* 2016;31:597–606.

19. Nelson SM. Prevention and management of ovarian hyperstimulation syndrome. *Thrombosis Res.* 2017;151(suppl 1):S61–S64.

20. Kramer W, Schneider J, Schultz N. US oocyte donors: A retrospective study of medical and psychosocial issues. *Human Reprod.* 2009;24:3144–9.

21. Ahuja K, Simons E. Cancer of the colon in an egg donor: Policy repercussions for donor recruitment. *Human Reprod.* 1998;13:227–8.

22. Schneider J. Fatal colon cancer in a young egg donor: A physician mother's call for follow-up and research on the long-term risks of ovarian stimulation. *Fertil Steril.* 2008;90:1–5.

23. Kenney N, McGowan M. Looking back: Egg donors' retrospective evaluations of their motivations, expectations, and experiences during their first donation cycle. *Fertil Steril.* 2010;93:455–66.

24. Jordan C, Belar C, Williams S. Anonymous oocyte donation: A follow-up analysis of donors' experiences. *J Psychosom Obstet Gynecol.* 2004;25:145–51.

25. Ethics Committee of the American Society of Reproductive Medicine. Informing offspring of their conception by gamete or embryo donation: A committee opinion. *Fertil Steril.* 2013;100:45–9.

26. Talladini M, Zanchettin L, Gronchi G, Morsan V. Parental disclosure of assisted reproductive technology (ART) conception to their children: A systematic and meta-analytic review. *Human Reprod.* 2016;31:1275–87.

27. Soderstrom-Anttila V, Salevaara M, Suikkari A. Increasing openness in oocyte donation families regarding disclosure over 15 years. *Human Reprod.* 2010;25:2535–42.

28. Greenfeld D, Klock S. Disclosure decisions among known and anonymous oocyte donation recipients. *Fertil Steril.* 2004;81:1565–71.

29. Hahn S, Craft-Rosenberg M. The disclosure decisions of parents who conceive children using donor eggs. *J Obstet Gynecol Neonatal Nurs.* 2002;31:283–93.

30. Golombok S, Murray C, Brinsden P, Abdall H. Social versus biological parenting: Family functioning and the socioemotional development of children conceived by egg or sperm donation. *J Child Psychol Psychiatry.* 1999;40:519–27.

31. Murray C, MacCallum F, Golombok S. Egg donation parents and their children: Follow-up at age 12 years. *Fertil Steril.* 2006;85:610–18.

32. Bos H, van Balen F. Children of the new reproductive technologies: Social and genetic parenthood. *Patient Educ Counsel.* 2010;81:429–35.

33. Blyth E, Cranshaw M, Frith L, Jones C. Donor-conceived people's views and experiences of their genetic origins: A critical analysis of the research evidence. *J Law Med.* 2012;19:769–80.

34. Zweifel J. Donor conception from the viewpoint of the child: Positives, negatives, and promoting the welfare of the child. *Fertil Steril.* 2015;104:513–19.

35. Ravelingien A, Provoost V, Pennings G. Open-identity sperm donation: How does offering donor-identifying information related to donor-conceived offspring's wishes and needs? *Bioethical Inquiry.* 2015;12:503–9.

36. Braverman A, Schlaff WD. End of anonymity: Stepping into the dawn of communication and a new paradigm in gamete donor counseling. *Fertil Steril.* 2019;111:1102–4.

9

Oncofertility

Ethics and Hope after Cancer

*Bruno Ramalho de Carvalho MD, MSc, MBA, Jhenifer Kliemchen
Rodrigues BSc, MSc, PhD, and Teresa K. Woodruff PhD*

Introduction

Advances in cancer treatment, particularly chemotherapeutics, are expected to lead to significant improvements in survival rates. Indeed, the last report of the American Cancer Society (ACS), the Centers for Disease Control and Prevention (CDC), the National Cancer Institute (NCI), and the North American Association of Central Cancer Registries (NAACCR) estimates an overall decrease of 0.6% per year in cancer incidence rates from 2012 to 2016, and an average decrease of 1.5% per year in cancer death rates from 2013 to 2017. Among children and adolescents, respectively, cancer incidence rates increased an average of 0.8% and 0.9% per year from 2012 to 2016, and cancer deaths decreased an average of 1.4% and 1.0%.[1]

While cancer incidence and death rates are decreasing, quality of life after cancer may still be reduced due to early functional failure of the gonads and, consequently, infertility, resulting from either the disease itself or its treatment. Unfortunately, it is difficult to quantify or qualify the occurrence of gonadotoxic damage and to assess whether the eventual damage will lead to definitive gonadal dysfunction.[2] In this context, questions and proposals arise for improving and maintaining the quality of life after cancer, among which are strategies for the preservation of gonadal function and/or gametes, and, therefore, the preservation of chances of having genetic descendants and even of being able to carry a pregnancy.

For that purpose, oncofertility is an interdisciplinary field that bridges oncology and reproductive endocrinology to address the quality of life issues that concern young cancer patients whose fertility may be threatened by their disease or its treatment.[3] Oncofertility requires a cross-disciplinary interaction between a number of different stakeholders, including physicians, basic scientists, clinical researchers, nurses, psychologists, ethicists, lawyers, educators, and religious leaders. As with any discipline under development, oncofertility is currently undergoing a period of maturation and transformation in which ethical and bioethical questions weigh heavily.

This chapter gives a brief background of fertility preservation in the cancer setting—oncofertility—provides context for bioethics, and explores the ethical dilemmas associated with oncofertility practice, including safety, efficacy, informed consent/assent, tissue storage, and posthumous reproduction.

Fertility Preservation in the Cancer Setting: Oncofertility

There are many options and techniques available for the preservation of gametes in men, women, and children. Each patient is unique: the impact of a given treatment on fertility can vary and so can the time available before starting lifesaving treatments. Patient age and pubertal status, marital status, personal wishes, religious and cultural constraints, and prognosis may all affect decision-making. Fertility preservation must be tailored to the individual circumstances and integrated with the treatment regimen. Close coordination between the treating physician and the reproductive endocrinologist is the key to preserving family-building options for patients.

For men, fertility preservation options may include sperm banking, gonadal shielding, testicular sperm extraction (TESE), and testicular tissue cryopreservation. For women, embryo banking, egg (oocyte) banking, ovarian tissue cryopreservation (experimental), radiation shielding, and ovarian transposition may be options. While many of these options are already considered standard of care and used routinely, others are still considered experimental. In both instances, ethical issues on the subject are still being debated. The remainder of this chapter will explore the ethics of oncofertility.

Fertility Preservation: Medical or Social Motivations?

There is a unique duality involved in confronting a life-threatening diagnosis while simultaneously considering the human desire to have a child.

This duality presents a struggle both for patients with cancer and for clinicians.[4] There is no doubt that one of the greatest benefits of fertility preservation is emotional, since the impossibility of biological procreation may generate anguish, sharpen feelings of impotence in the face of cancer, and even lead to family and social life disorders.[5] From the medical point of view, it should be made clear to the patient that the temporary or permanent absence of endocrine and reproductive functions after anti-cancer treatment depends on variables such as location of the disease, therapeutic regimen used, doses administered, route of administration, and age of the person at the time of gonadotoxic treatment.[6,7] Considering such variables, children and adolescents may experience less severe changes in gonadal function.[8]

However, providing options to preserve fertility can help to achieve the goal of optimizing quality of life for cancer survivors, particularly those affected by the disease prior to having children. Social motivation here is the strongest point. However, while acknowledging the merits of social impact, questions arise since, from a technical point of view, individuals are not necessarily infertile at the time of cancer treatment or will be infertile after its completion.[9] Moreover, concerns about the health risks of hormonal administration and anti-cancer treatment delay are not supported by literature.[10] Finally, although there are limited data on the safety of ovarian stimulation in women with cancer, observational studies taken more than ten years of follow-up after breast cancer suggest there is no impact over disease-free survival,[11-15] at least among those who were treated with aromatase inhibitors co-administration.[16]

Ethics and Bioethics

Although there may be some conflict between social and medical positioning, the provision of strategies aiming to preserve reproductive capacity in the face of any type of treatment that may harm it becomes a moral obligation and respects the autonomy of choices, which is an essential foundation for a free society.[17]

To gain a better understanding of ethical dilemmas in oncofertility, some general background on bioethics is necessary. Traditionally, the framework of analysis of ethical issues in medicine uses four principles, which were mentioned preliminarily in the Belmont Report[18] and had their use consecrated by Beauchamp and Childress[19] as pillars for establishing limits to clinical practice and research:

- *Autonomy*: Respect for the individual, his or her own convictions, judgments, and choices, and protection for those with diminished autonomy; in the context of assisted reproductive technologies (ART) and oncofertility, all choices are recommended to be duly recorded in an informed consent form.
- *Beneficence*: Promoting well-being, from maximizing benefits and minimizing harm to the individual; in the context of ART and oncofertility, it should be respected by offering strategies to avoid the inability to procreate as a consequence of anti-neoplastic treatments, assuming that the possibility of forming a family is part of the best interest of cancer survivors.
- *Justice*: Equitable, impartial treatment based on equal opportunities; in the context of ART and oncofertility, it contemplates universal access.
- *Nonmaleficence*: Obligation not to impose risks or cause harm to the individual; in the scope of ART and oncofertility, it supports the selection of the safest ovulation induction protocol, including strategies to avoid the growth of hormonal-dependent tumors.

Additionally, the advent of new technologies and the advancing knowledge on treatment of diseases once considered fatal, such as cancer, prompts the renewal of ethical and philosophical concepts about the interference of medicine and related areas on the human body, its well-being and integrity. It is in this context that bioethics emerges.

Bioethics establishes principles of conduct based on traditional values and broadens their horizon by promoting the analysis of issues related to medicine and life sciences, by both adopting new technologies and their alternative forms of application and by taking into account their social, legal, and environmental dimensions.[20] It emerges in the scenario of a growing awareness of the great transformations in the spheres of science, economics, and law, which have had a profound impact on social life since the second half of the twentieth century.[21] In the context of bioethics applied to oncofertility, the intersections of the biological, psychosocial, and economic aspects lead to concerns that touch on ART, reproductive rights, and the freedom of choice for people with cancer and ultimately refer to the safety of the patient and their intended offspring.

Oncofertility, Safety, and Effectiveness

While many fertility preservation options are considered standard of care, some fertility preservation procedures available to both men and women are still considered experimental and naturally there are concerns with the safety of these procedures. The next two sections explore the safety and effectiveness of oncofertility practices, including those procedures that are still considered experimental.

Cryopreservation of Gametes

Cryopreservation of gametes is currently considered the strategy of choice for fertility preservation in people with cancer,[22] because it is effective for both males and females, and it eliminates the ethical, legal, and religious dilemmas involved in the freezing of embryos, especially in view of the possibility of short survival of cancer patients, but also when the disease affects adolescents, single people, or those who, for personal reasons, are against the freezing of embryos. Of note, fertility preservation interventions should be offered as early as possible, preferably before treatment starts.[23]

Males

Sperm cryopreservation is the only well-established and effective strategy for postpubertal male candidates who receive cancer treatment. Indeed, hormonal gonadoprotection is ineffective for men, and other methods, such as testicular tissue cryopreservation for future reimplantation or grafting, are considered experimental and should be performed only as part of approved research protocols.[23]

Females

The evolution of knowledge about the vitrification and warming of human mature oocytes has been growing in past decades, and it is expected that more than 85% of cryopreserved gametes survive the process.[24] According to the literature, the respective rates of fertilization, clinical pregnancy, and live births using frozen gametes are approximately 70%, 57%, and 39%, respectively,[24] which are close to the results for fresh gametes.

From an ethical point of view, an important issue in oocyte cryopreservation has been the need to postpone anti-neoplastic treatment, thus compromising prognosis. However, with the development of random-start treatment protocols that are independent of the menstrual cycle and allow the capture of oocytes in about two weeks (postponing the beginning of cancer treatment only for this period), this is no longer a pressing concern. Also, the addition of an aromatase inhibitor or a selective estrogen receptor modulator to an ovarian stimulation protocol is now well-established and may mitigate concerns about the prognosis of estrogen-sensitive breast and gynecologic malignancies; studies do not indicate increased cancer recurrence risk as a result of ovarian stimulation with this hormonal protection.[10,23,25-27]

Ovarian tissue cryopreservation aimed at future transplantation has recently been considered no longer experimental by the American Society for Reproductive Medicine, presenting a live birth rate of 29% after reimplantation.[28,29] The intervention carries the advantages of not requiring ovarian stimulation and being an immediate intervention. Furthermore, it is the only option which may restore global ovarian function, does not require pubertal status, and is the only method acceptable for patients who are children. However, the possibility of metastasis reimplantation is a matter of concern, and robust data confirming its safety for some tumors, like leukemias, are not available to date.[23,30]

Ovarian suppression by gonadotropin-releasing hormone agonists (GnRHa) or other means is supported by conflicting evidence and should not be used in place of oocyte, embryo, or ovarian tissue cryopreservation. Indeed, GnRHa may be offered if those proven effective methods are not feasible[23] or as a complementary intervention after them and before anticancer treatment initiation.

No less important are the possible surgical interventions intending to preserve fertility in women with cancer. Beyond fertility-sparing surgical approaches, ovarian transposition can be offered to patient candidates of pelvic irradiation, but women should be aware that the intervention is not always successful because of radiation scatter or the possibility of ovarian repositioning[23] and because it does not protect the gonads from chemotherapy, which is commonly associated with radiotherapy.

Finally, there are few reports documenting the possibility of aspirating oocytes from surgically removed ovaries, either immature[31-36] or mature,[37–40] thus supporting the offer of fertility preservation to ovarian cancer patients while mitigating the risk of malignant cell spillage.

Informed Consent for Young Adult Cancer Patients

Informed consent is the bedrock of work in emerging reproductive technologies and ensures that the patient and the practitioner are aware of the boundary conditions associated with medical interventions. In the case of cancer patients, provision of the best and most recent information about the potential risks and the currently available interventions for the preservation of their reproductive functions allows them to make the right decisions with the necessary clarity, based on personal interests and perspectives.[41]

Pediatric and Adolescent Assent

Complex ethical situations are involved in fertility preservation strategies for children, namely a lack of understanding of those aspects that refer to sexuality, a desire for children in the distant future, and the need for ART for future procreation with their own gametes or gonadal tissues; the assumption of the desire for procreation or the psychosocial trauma from infertility in adult life; and the inherent risks from invasive procedures involved in the preservation of gametes or gonadal tissues.[42–45] Furthermore, guidance about future reproductive health must be carefully discussed in a manner coherent with cognitive status of the child.[46]

Although there is not a clear moment when children become sufficiently mature for informed consent or refusal, children older than seven years must be encouraged to opine about their interests in general future health, even if such positions are contrary to the desire of the parents.[47,48] However, it is illusory to expect an absolutely voluntary choice in any decision-making process related to health issues from a child or an adolescent. In such patients, autonomy may be incomplete, and parents' opinions may influence, at least in part, the final decision for any consent or refusal.[46]

In the majority of cases, parents are the appropriate surrogate medical decision-makers for their children and adolescents, based on the intimate understanding of their social and emotional needs and family values. Thus oncofertility facilities must develop thoughtful guidance from the physician and the whole interdisciplinary health team, in an attempt to (1) share information in a continuous physician-patient-family communication and education process, (2) educate patients sufficiently to enable them to make an informed decision to consent or decline, (3) mitigate as much as possible the risks of any harm; and (4) respect the ethical and legal aspects in each country.[46]

Case Study

To address the most problematic ethical issues of fertility preservation in cancer patients, a hypothetical case is explored here. As an exercise for the reader, we briefly highlight possible implications of fertility preservation in cancer patients. The previously mentioned concepts can serve as a theoretical background for clinicians facing complex situations and ethical concerns and to reinforce arguments to support or reject available strategies.

The case involves a 24-year-old university student. She does not have any immediate plans to have children at present, but she does hope to have children in the future. Two weeks ago, she was diagnosed with breast cancer and now needs to schedule chemotherapy, which may leave her infertile. While she is confident about treatment success, she is troubled by the possibility that treatment might impair her ability to have children. Her oncologist has already informed her that she is a candidate egg freezing, but that this decision needs to be made within two weeks.

The implications of oocyte cryopreservation, while interrelated and intertwined, may be grouped for didactic purposes into medical, financial, psychosocial, legal-ethical, and relational.[49]

Medical implications: If she opts for oocyte cryopreservation, the retrieval strategy includes ovarian stimulation with gonadotropins followed by vaginal egg retrieval, which can be complicated by minor bleeding. Adverse effects such as ovarian hyperstimulation syndrome must be taken into consideration, mainly in women at high risk, such as those with polycystic ovarian syndrome. It must also be noted that cryopreserved oocytes do not guarantee a future pregnancy and that in vitro fertilization (IVF) will be necessary for reproductive success if the preserved gametes are needed.

Financial implications: Oocyte freezing costs vary depending on the country and on the patient's needs. It is important to note that costs are not limited to procedure retrieval and storage expenses, but also include IVF costs and eventual supernumerary embryo cryopreservation.

Psychosocial implications: People rarely consider that they might need to undergo fertility preservation until they are faced with an unanticipated situation. In these cases, decisions must often be made with strict time constraints. The potential for infertility resulting from medical treatment often generates anguish and a feeling of impotence, which adds to the emotional load of the underlying disease itself. But, from a purely technical view, it is not predictable whether cancer patients will become infertile as a result of their cancer treatments.[9] Thus, accepting or rejecting fertility preservation, as does offering strategies for it, transits through moral obligation and challenges the right for autonomy.

Legal-ethical implications: The most problematic aspects of gamete cryopreservation from a legal and ethical standpoint are the status of gamete ownership, posthumous use, and the possibility of discarding or donating gametes to research or to a third party.

Relational implications: Relational implications mainly involve the support and expectations of people with significant relations to the cryopreserved material. The possibility of pressure to pursue procreation may override personal preferences.

The Role of Professional Societies and Organizations

It is important for any clinician or oncofertility health professional to stay up to date with clinical guidelines. Knowledge and understanding of guidelines from professional societies including the American Society of Clinical Oncology (ASCO), the American Society of Reproductive Medicine (ASRM), the American Society of Pediatrics (ASP), the American Association of Urological (AAU), the British Fertility Society, the European Society of Human Reproduction and Embryology (ESRHE), and the International Society for Fertility Preservation (ISFP) are an important part in providing clinical oncofertility care to patients. These guidelines are necessary to the appropriate vetting process and present well-tested and standardized interventions for practitioners. Standard methods for males are sperm banking, while the experimental intervention is testicular tissue freezing or transposition. For females, standard methods include embryo and oocyte freezing, ovarian transposition with experimental/alternative methods to include ovarian tissue cryopreservation, and ovarian suppression.[4,50] The guidelines are very similar and in general state that, as part of education and informed consent before cancer therapy, oncologists should address the possibility of infertility and be prepared to discuss possible fertility preservation options or refer appropriate and interested patients to reproductive specialists. Clinical judgment should be employed in the timing of raising this issue, but discussion at the earliest possible opportunity is encouraged. Several studies show that less than half of oncologists who participated in a survey project routinely referred reproductive-aged cancer patients to fertility specialists.[51]

Professional societies and other organizations work together to convene the field of oncofertility in order to accelerate the pace and improve the quality of oncofertility research and practice.[50] Established in 2007, the Oncofertility Consortium at Northwestern University is an international, interdisciplinary initiative designed to explore the reproductive future of cancer survivors. Some patients may be interested in participating in scientific research involving experimental fertility preservation techniques, including ovarian tissue cryopreservation and testicular tissue cryopreservation. To assist, the Oncofertility Consortium provides templates of institutional review board (IRB) forms that can be downloaded and copied for organizations or individual practices that wish to seek approval at local sites. These templates can be found online at www.oncofertility.northwestern.edu.

In addition, the Oncofertility Consortium and other fertility preservation organizations suggest conversations about alternative family-building options including donor sperm, donor eggs, surrogacy, or adoption, although these third-party options are not available in all countries or contexts.[52] To aid in the conversation, the Oncofertility Consortium provides tools to enable thoughtful, deliberative, consent-based engagement. In the end, the patients' medical condition and wishes are most important to the procedures offered.

Final Considerations

Post-treatment fertility has emerged as an important issue in the early counseling of individuals with cancer since survivors may have their quality of life affected by the functional failure of the gonads secondary to antineoplastic therapies. In this context, oncofertility has been developed as an interdisciplinary field of study that combines expertise in reproductive medicine and oncology to provide strategies aiming to maintain the possibility of future procreation. Today, many options and techniques are available for the preservation of gametes in men and women. Some of these techniques are already considered well-established and are used routinely, but ethical and moral issues on the subject must still be debated.[41]

As the field continues to develop, there are several areas in which our practice has improved. However, several ethical concerns still exist involving beneficence, nonmaleficence, informed consent, adolescent assent, and posthumous use of reproductive tissues. Because the field is still developing, great disparities exist in available options depending on age, ability to pay, and geographic location. Such discrepancies in access may lead to health disparities in the patient population. As the science continues to make future fertility more feasible, the ethical questions will continue to become more complex.[53]

Additional Resources

The Oncofertility Consortium: www.oncofertility.northwestern.edu
SaveMyFertility.org
Preservefertility.northwestern.edu
American Society for Reproductive Medicine
American Society of Clinical Oncology
European Society of Human Reproduction and Embryology

Acknowledgments

The authors gratefully acknowledge Lauren Ataman for her editorial assistance on this work.

References

1. Henley SJ, Ward EM, Scott S, et al. Annual report to the nation on the status of cancer, part I: National cancer statistics. *Cancer.* 2020;126(10):2225–49.
2. Deepinder F, Agarwal A. Technical and ethical challenges of fertility preservation in young cancer patients. *Reprod Biomed Online.* 2008;16(6):784–91.

3. Woodruff TK. The emergence of a new interdiscipline: Oncofertility. *Cancer Treat Res.* 2007;138:3–11.

4. Jeruss JS, Woodruff TK. Preservation of fertility in patients with cancer. *N Engl J Med.* 2009;360(9):902–11.

5. Dudzinski DM. Ethical issues in fertility preservation for adolescent cancer survivors: Oocyte and ovarian tissue cryopreservation. *J Pediatr Adolesc Gynecol.* 2004;17(2):97–102.

6. Pentheroudakis G, Orecchia R, Hoekstra HJ, Pavlidis N. ESMO Guidelines Working Group. Cancer, fertility and pregnancy: ESMO clinical practice guidelines for diagnosis, treatment and follow-up. *Ann Oncol.* 2010;21(suppl 5):v266–273.

7. Christinat A, Pagani O. Fertility after breast cancer. *Maturitas.* 2012;73(3):191–6.

8. Rosa-e-Silva ACJS, Rosa-e-Silva JC, Reis RM, Tone LG, Sá MFS, Ferriani RA. Gonadal function in adolescent patients submitted to chemotherapy during childhood or during the pubertal period. *J Pediatr Adolesc Gynecol.* 2007;20(2):89–91.

9. Basco D, Campo-Engelstein L, Rodriguez S. Insuring against infertility: Expanding state infertility mandates to include fertility preservation technology for cancer patients. *J Law Med Ethics.* 2010;38(4):832–39.

10. Letourneau JM, Sinha N, Wald K, et al. Random start ovarian stimulation for fertility preservation appears unlikely to delay initiation of neoadjuvant chemotherapy for breast cancer. *Hum Reprod.* 2017;32(10):2123–9.

11. Azim AA, Costantini-Ferrando M, Oktay K. Safety of fertility preservation by ovarian stimulation with letrozole and gonadotropins in patients with breast cancer: A prospective controlled study. *J Clin Oncol.* 2008;26(16):2630–35.

12. Turan V, Bedoschi G, Moy F, Oktay K. Safety and feasibility of performing two consecutive ovarian stimulation cycles with the use of letrozole-gonadotropin protocol for fertility preservation in breast cancer patients. *Fertil Steril.* 2013;100(6):1681–5.e1.

13. Meirow D, Raanani H, Maman E, et al. Tamoxifen co-administration during controlled ovarian hyperstimulation for in vitro fertilization in breast cancer patients increases the safety of fertility-preservation treatment strategies. *Fertil Steril.* 2014;102(2):488–95.e3.

14. Kim J, Turan V, Oktay K. Long-term safety of letrozole and gonadotropin stimulation for fertility preservation in women with breast cancer. *J Clin Endocrinol Metab.* 2016;101(4):1364–71.

15. Rodriguez-Wallberg KA, Eloranta S, Krawiec K, Lissmats A, Bergh J, Liljegren A. Safety of fertility preservation in breast cancer patients in a register-based matched cohort study. *Breast Cancer Res Treat.* 2018;167(3):761–9.

16. Rodgers RJ, Reid GD, Koch J, et al. The safety and efficacy of controlled ovarian hyperstimulation for fertility preservation in women with early breast cancer: A systematic review. *Hum Reprod.* 2017;32(5):1033–45.

17. Larcher V. The ethical obligation to preserve fertility in the face of all therapies that might adversely affect it. *Arch Dis Child.* 2012;97(9):767–68.

18. Baier K. Ethical principles and their validity. The National Commission for the Protection of Human Subjects of Biomedical and Behavioral Research. Belmont Report: Ethical Principles and Guidelines for the Protection of Human Subjects of Research, Appendix, Volume I, 1978. Retrieved from https://videocast.nih.gov/pdf/ohrp_appendix_belmont_report_vol_1.pdf

19. Beauchamp TL, Childress JF. Principles of Biomedical Ethics. 5th ed. New York: Oxford University Press; 2001.

20. United Nations Educational, Scientific and Cultural Organization (UNESCO). *Universal Declaration on Bioethics and Human Rights*. Paris: Unesco; 2005. Retrieved fromhttp://portal.unesco.org/en/ev.php-URL_ID=31058&URL_DO=DO_TOPIC&URL_SECTION=201.html

21. Selli L, Garrafa V. Bioethics, critical solidarity and organic volunteering. *Rev Saude Publica*. 2005;39(3):473–8.

22. Loren AW, Mangu PB, Beck LN, et al. Fertility preservation for patients with cancer: American Society of Clinical Oncology clinical practice guideline update. *J Clin Oncol*. 2013;31(19):2500–10.

23. Oktay K, Harvey BE, Partridge AH, et al. Fertility preservation in patients with cancer: ASCO clinical practice guideline update. *J Clin Oncol*. 2018;36(19): 1994–2001.

24. Doyle JO, Richter KS, Lim J, Stillman RJ, Graham JR, Tucker MJ. Successful elective and medically indicated oocyte vitrification and warming for autologous in vitro fertilization, with predicted birth probabilities for fertility preservation according to number of cryopreserved oocytes and age at retrieval. *Fertil Steril*. 2016;105(2):459–66.e2.

25. Franco JG Jr, Oliveira JB, Petersen CG, Mauri AL, Baruffi R, Cavagna M. Adjuvant therapy with GnRH agonists/tamoxifen in breast cancer should be a good council for patients with hormone receptor-positive tumours and wish to preserve fertility. *Med Hypotheses*. 2012;78(4):442–5.

26. Cakmak H, Katz A, Cedars MI, Rosen MP. Effective method for emergency fertility preservation: Random-start controlled ovarian stimulation. *Fertil Steril*. 2013;100(6):1673–80.

27. Cakmak H, Rosen MP. Ovarian stimulation in cancer patients. *Fertil Steril*. 2013;99(6):1476–84.

28. Donnez J, Dolmans MM, Diaz C, Pellicer A. Ovarian cortex transplantation: Time to move on from experimental studies to open clinical application. *Fertil Steril*. 2015;104(5):1097–8.

29. Jensen AK, Macklon KT, Fedder J, Ernst E, Humaidan P, Andersen CY. 86 successful births and 9 ongoing pregnancies worldwide in women transplanted with frozen-thawed ovarian tissue: Focus on birth and perinatal outcome in 40 of these children. *J Assist Reprod Genet*. 2017;34(3):325–36.

30. Jensen AK, Kristensen SG, Macklon KT, et al. Outcomes of transplantations of cryopreserved ovarian tissue to 41 women in Denmark. *Hum Reprod*. 2015;30(12): 2838–45.

31. Revel A, Safran A, Benshushan A, Shushan A, Laufer N, Simon A. In vitro maturation and fertilization of oocytes from an intact ovary of a surgically treated patient with endometrial carcinoma: Case report. *Hum Reprod*. 2004;19(7):1608–11.

32. Huang JY, Buckett WM, Gilbert L, Tan SL, Chian RC. Retrieval of immature oocytes followed by in vitro maturation and vitrification: A case report on a new strategy of fertility preservation in women with borderline ovarian malignancy. *Gynecol Oncol*. 2007;105(2):542–4.

33. Fadini R, Dal Canto M, Mignini Renzini M, et al. Embryo transfer following in vitro maturation and cryopreservation of oocytes recovered from antral follicles during conservative surgery for ovarian cancer. *J Assist Reprod Genet*. 2012;29(8):779–81.

34. Prasath EB, Chan ML, Wong WH, et al. First pregnancy and live birth resulting from cryopreserved embryos obtained from in vitro matured oocytes after oophorectomy in an ovarian cancer patient. *Hum Reprod.* 2014;29(2):276–8.

35. Segers I, Mateizel I, Van Moer E, et al. In vitro maturation (IVM) of oocytes recovered from ovariectomy specimens in the laboratory: A promising "ex vivo" method of oocyte cryopreservation resulting in the first report of an ongoing pregnancy in Europe. *J Assist Reprod Genet.* 2015;32(8):1221–31.

36. Park CW, Lee SH, Yang KM, et al. Cryopreservation of in vitro matured oocytes after ex vivo oocyte retrieval from gynecologic cancer patients undergoing radical surgery. *Clín Exp Reproducers Med.* 2016;43(2):119–25.

37. Fatemi HM, Kyrou D, Al-Azemi M, et al. Ex-vivo oocyte retrieval for fertility preservation. *Fertil Steril.* 2011;95(5):1787.e15–e17.

38. Bocca S, Dedmond D, Jones E, Stadtmauer L, Oehninger S. Successful extracorporeal mature oocyte harvesting after laparoscopic oophorectomy following controlled ovarian hyperstimulation for the purpose of fertility preservation in a patient with borderline ovarian tumor. *J Assist Reprod Genet.* 2011;28(9):771–2.

39. Pereira N, Hubschmann AG, Lekovich JP, Schattman GL, Rosenwaks Z. Ex vivo retrieval and cryopreservation of oocytes from oophorectomized specimens for fertility preservation in a BRCA1 mutation carrier with ovarian cancer. *Fertil Steril.* 2017;108(2):357–60.

40. de la Blanca EP, Fernandez-Perez MF, Martin-Diaz EDM, Lozano M, Garcia-Sanchez M, Monedero C. Ultrasound-guided *ex-vivo* retrieval of mature oocytes for fertility preservation during laparoscopic oophorectomy: A case report. *J Reprod Infertil.* 2018;19(3):174–81.

41. Carvalho BR, Kliemchen J, Woodruff TK. Ethical, moral and other aspects related to fertility preservation in cancer patients. *JBRA Assist Reprod.* 2017;21(1):45–8.

42. Gracia CR, Gracia JJE, Chen S. Ethical dilemmas in oncofertility: An exploration of three clinical scenarios. *Cancer Treat Res.* 2010;156:195–208.

43. Patrizio P, Caplan AL. Ethical issues surrounding fertility preservation in cancer patients. *Clin Obstet Gynecol* 2010;53:717–26.

44. Joshi S, Savani BN, Chow EJ, et al. Clinical guide to fertility preservation in hematopoietic cell transplant recipients. *Bone Marrow Transplant.* 2014;49(4):477–84.

45. McDougall RJ, Gillam L, Delany C, Jayasinghe Y. Ethics of fertility preservation for prepubertal children: Should clinicians offer procedures where efficacy is largely unproven? *J Med Ethics.* 2018;44(1):27–31.

46. Katz AL, Webb SA. Committee on Bioethics. Informed consent in decision-making in pediatric practice. *Pediatrics.* 2016;138(2):e20161484.

47. American Academy of Pediatrics, Committee on Bioethics. Informed consent, parental permission, and assent in pediatric practice. *Pediatrics.* 1995;95:314–17.

48. Shah DK, Goldman E, Fisseha S. Medical, ethical, and legal considerations in fertility preservation. *Int J Gynecol Obstet* 2011;115:11–15.

49. Linkeviciute A, Boniolo G, Chiavari L, Peccatori FA. Fertility preservation in cancer patients: the global framework. *Cancer Treat Rev.* 2014 Sep;40(8):1019–27. doi:10.1016/j.ctrv.2014.06.001. Epub 2014 Jun 11. PMID: 24953980.

50. Ataman LM, Rodrigues JK, Marinho RM, et al. Creating a global community of practice for oncofertility. *J Glob Oncol.* 2016;2(2):83–96.

51. Köhler TS, Kondapalli LA, Shah A, Chan A, Woodruff TK, Brannigan RE. Results from the survey for preservation of adolescent reproduction (SPARE) study: Gender disparity in delivery of fertility preservation message to adolescents with cancer. *J Assist Reprod Genet.* 2011;28(3):269–77.

52. Rashedi AS, Roo SF, Ataman LM, et al. Survey of third-party parenting options associated with fertility preservation available to patients with cancer around the globe. *J Global Oncol.* 2018:4:1–7.

53. Runco DV, Taylor JF, Helft PR. Ethical Barriers in Adolescent Oncofertility Counseling. *J Pediatr Hematol Oncol.* 2017;39(1):56–61.

Suggested Readings

Council of Europe, European Convention for the Protection of Human Rights and Fundamental Freedoms, as amended by Protocols Nos. 11 and 14, 4 November 1950, ETS 5. Retrieved from http://www.refworld.org/docid/3ae6b3b04.html

Ferlay J, Soerjomataram I, Dikshit R, et al. Cancer incidence and mortality worldwide: Sources, methods and major patterns in GLOBOCAN 2012. *Int J Cancer.* 2015;136(5):E359–86.

Jemal A, Center MM, DeSantis C, Ward EM. Global patterns of cancer incidence and mortality rates and trends. *Cancer Epidemiol Biomarkers Prev.* 2010;19(8):1893–1907.

Leroy F. Human rights and procreation. *Rev Med Brux.* 1990;11(4):83–88.

Torre LA, Bray F, Siegel RL, Ferlay J, Lortet-Tieulent J, Jemal A. Global cancer statistics, 2012. *Cancer J Clin.* 2015;65(2):87–108.

UN General Assembly. International Covenant on Civil and Political Rights, 16 December 1966, United Nations, Treaty Series, vol. 999, p.171. Retrieved from http://www.refworld.org/docid/3ae6b3aa0.html

UN General Assembly. Universal Declaration of Human Rights, 10 December 1948, 217 A (III). Retrieved fromhttp://www.refworld.org/docid/3ae6b3712c.html

UN Population Fund (UNFPA). Report of the International Conference on Population and Development, Cairo, 5–13 September 1994, 1995, A/CONF.171/13/Rev.1. Retrieved fromhttp://www.refworld.org/docid/4a54bc080.html

UN Population Fund (UNFPA). Report of the International Conference on Population and Development, Cairo, 5–13 September 1994, 1995, A/CONF.171/13/Rev.1. Retrieved fromhttp://www.refworld.org/docid/4a54bc080.html

Woodruff TK, Clayman M, Walmey KE. *Oncofertility Communication: Sharing Information and Building Relationships Across Disciplines.* 1st ed. New York: Springer; 2014.

10

Accessing Reproductive Technology in France

Strengths and Limits of a Model that Privileges "Just Reproduction" above Respect for Autonomy

Laurence Brunet MLS and Véronique Fournier MD, PhD

While access to all kinds of reproductive technologies has always been possible in the United States, at least for those who are wealthy enough to afford it, in France providing assisted reproductive technologies (ART) remains strictly regulated. Until 2020, it was legally forbidden for a lesbian couple or a single woman to access sperm insemination.[1] And as for surrogacy, the 2020 law does not change the previous regulation: it remains strictly forbidden to use it either for a heterosexual or homosexual couple. In contrast to the American model that maximizes the value of individual autonomy, the French model has historically been to prioritize the respect of collective values. As such, for example, in the French perspective, the organization of ART must respect the principle of noncommodification of the human body—meaning that removal or transfer of any part of the body must be noncommercial and associated with the principle of full collective and financial solidarity vis-à-vis any medical/therapeutic need of patients—meaning that the state pays for almost all the treatments any patient needs, including access to ART. In brief, it can be said that France privileges "just reproduction" and strict state regulation of ART activity, whereas the United States promotes the respect of reproductive autonomy for individuals and the liberal organization of reproductive practices.[2] In this chapter, we further describe the conditions for obtaining ART in France, which appears as a counterexample to the American approach. We first give some concrete examples of what is or is not possible in terms of access to ART in France, then detail the main arguments on which the French law relies to highlight how healthcare systems are products of choices and cultures rather than accident. Finally, we discuss the model on its ethical merits and stress its limits from an ethical point of view.

Access to ART in France

Until now, access to ART in France was only authorized as a "medical response to a medical problem."[3] As such, this access was quite restrictive compared to other models. But, in contrast, all people who were granted access to ART in France were financially covered by public funds. We further detail later these two main aspects of the French ART model.

Restrictive Access

The previous French bioethics law stated that ART "seeks to remedy the infertility of a couple, or prevent the transmission of a particularly serious illness from a member of the couple to the child" (article L. 2141-2 of the Code de la Santé Publique or Code of Public Health (CSP)). It insisted that "the pathological nature of [the patient's] infertility" must be "medically diagnosed." Furthermore, since ART in France served to alleviate the anatomic or physiologic inability to procreate naturally, access to ART was only possible for heterosexual couples. Other criteria included that the two members of the couple must be of child-bearing age and alive, thereby prohibiting all postmortem reproduction (article L 2141-2 al. 2 of the CSP).[4]

This framework was supposed to ensure the child's best interest: a family unit built by his or her (two) heterosexual parents was considered to be the most suitable structure within which to raise a child. Indeed, the French law considered that it was in the child's best interest to have "a father and a mother, no more, no less."[5] Such requirements for accessing ART were supposed to foster the social acceptance of these techniques—which were accused, when they were introduced, of flouting the traditions of procreation founded on the biologic realities.[6] Moreover, the law gave, and still gives, the medical team a role of gatekeeper: the medical team can authorize, refuse, or postpone the access to ART in case of any doubt about the best interest of the unborn child.[7] As an example, we can cite an ethics consult we had some years ago: an ART team was strongly reluctant to give ART to a couple needing it for azoospermia, because both members of the couple were severely visually impaired and had a 50% risk of transmitting a mutation responsible for genetic bilateral aniridia and blindness to their baby. The parents had asked for in vitro fertilization with sperm donation and refused any prenatal diagnosis to check if the baby would inherit the mother's mutation. The healthcare team considered that the best interest of the future child could be challenged. The law gave them the discretionary power to refuse access to ART for this purpose. The ethics case conference on this case was very divided: some considered the parents were the most legitimate parties to decide and that to prevent them access could be likened to discrimination against those with disabilities; others were sensitive to the medical team's position, which worried about the birth of a baby with a disability, given that a lot of subsequent suffering for her and the whole family might have been avoided. Finally, after having postponed the decision during some long months and having conducted a thorough investigation into the social and psychological context of the family, the team decided to let this couple access ART. The baby was born with the mutation.

Generous Financial Coverage

In France, when access to ART is authorized, the process is implemented and universal health coverage pays 100% of the costs for all needed procedures (biological and clinical procedures, as well as full medication).[8] As such, although some limits are imposed on who can access full coverage,[9] France stands out among Western countries as the one with the most generous system of ART funding.

Those left out from ART Access

The ancient model of ART access precluded the use of ART for so-called social reasons of infertility (i.e., infertility due to sexual orientation or personal reasons). Undergoing ART in France for any purpose other than infertility stemming from medical etiologies risked severe punishment by the law, for both patients and doctors.[10] Consequently, those left out from ART access were numerous, and many of them decided to cross borders to obtain ART in foreign countries. Nevertheless, procreative relocations entailed some negative consequences, as in the example of lesbian couples and couples seeking surrogacy.

Families formed by gay and lesbian couples have only been very recently legally recognized in France (Same-Sex Marriage Law, May 17, 2013). For a lesbian couple in France, the most frequent way to start a family is through the use of sperm donation. The 2013 law authorizing same-sex marriage did not amend the framework of access to ART to allow lesbian couples to use it. Thus, until the recent law, the only option for lesbian couples who seek access to sperm donation remained to go abroad and pay for gametes to use in artificial insemination. Then, the second mother (the one who has not given birth) had to follow a judicial procedure to establish her maternity through adoption. This was a source of significant cost and stress, especially if the judge—as he or she had the right—ordered an investigation to ensure that the adoption was in the best interest of the child. For these reasons, increasing numbers of clinicians, scholars,[11] and public institutions have recently advocated for extending access to ART to lesbian couples, including, in June 2017, the French National Consultative Ethics Committee.[12]

As for families who have gone abroad for surrogacy, the consequences of the strict legislative conditions for access to ART in France remain onerous. Both traditional and gestational[13] surrogacies have been severely condemned in the French Civil Code since 1994.[14] So far no plan (with some exceptions[15]) has been made to soften the national stance on the illegality of surrogacy. However, cross-border surrogacy practices have expanded for infertile heterosexual parents and especially for gay couples, as a result of their recent legal recognition.[16] Once their children are born, parents bring them back to France and seek to have their foreign birth certificates transferred into French birth registers in order to achieve legal recognition of their parentage. Until 2014, the Court of Cassation, which is the supreme court of appeal in all civil and criminal cases, held a firm negative position on the matter: it persistently opposed the registration of foreign birth certificates and maintained that such an act was contrary to French public order and in contradiction with an essential principle of French law: the principle of the unavailability of personal status. This case law was challenged by the European Court of Human Rights (ECHR) in two rulings rendered on 26 June 2014 (*Labassée* and *Mennesson*[17]). According to the ECHR, the legal consequences of nonrecognition by French law of the relationship between children and intended parents "significantly affected the right to respect for private life, which implies that everyone must be able to establish the substance of his or her identity, including the legal parent–child relationship." Because ECHR decisions are binding in France since 1981, the country's courts became obliged to put an end to the contradictions existing between the national and European legal orders. It took three years after the EHCR rulings of 2014 to obtain the first case law reversal on the topic in France. In July 2017, a judge authorized a two-step process for intended parents to be registered as the legal parents on their child's birth certificate. First, only the biological parent is registered. Then, the second parent (the one with no biological link to the child; i.e., the intended mother or the second father) has to file a second-parent adoption request with a judge.

The Consistency and Strength of the French Bioethics Model

It is hard to understand France's approach concerning access to ART without taking into account the global bioethical legal framework that governs it. The goal of the first French law on bioethics, voted in 1994, was not only to regulate access to ART, but more largely to identify which common values should govern all medical uses of the human body. This led to the adoption of two laws on July 29, 1994,[18] which established a framework using a two-pronged approach. First, several new major principles concerning the respect of the human body were introduced into the Civil Code (chap. 8), with the intention that these founding principles remain unchanged and excluded from any subsequent revision of the second part of the legal framework, provided in the CSP. This second part established rules governing various biomedical practices, including access to ART, but with the idea that these regulations should be reviewed regularly to take into account scientific progress as well as significant societal evolutions.[19]

This double approach is intricately interwoven. As far as the respect of the human body is concerned, the French Civil Code provides, since 1994, fundamental principles that ensure "the primacy of the individual" and prohibit "any offense to the dignity of said individual" (Art. 16-1 c. civ). The rule stating that all surrogacy contracts are null and void is based on these foundations (Art. 16-7). Furthermore, the same code also details the norms regarding the non-ownership of the human body and, as mentioned earlier, the noncommodification of any part of the body that can be removed or transferred (Art. 16-5 and 16-6 c. civ). It is because of such norms that, for example, until 2020, donors remained strictly anonymous. The new law maintains the principle of anonymity at the time of sperm donation, but opens the possibility for a child to have access to the donor's identity under strict conditions. Moreover, the donor can't be financially rewarded for any body part (organ, tissue, cell, or gamete) donation.[20] The noncommodification of the human body implies that no one can pretend to directly pay for medical treatments where body or material parts are exchanged. However, when people are legally authorized to have access to such treatments, all costs are covered by public universal health coverage.

In France, the choice to privilege the organization of bioethics activities on reproductive justice, financial solidarity, and strict state regulation, rather than on respect for reproductive autonomy and liberal organization, led to the delegation of the control of the field, especially ART, to a national official health agency, the Agence de la Biomédecine(the ABM).[21] The ABM's mission is to authorize, evaluate, and regularly renew the certification of all services and departments that work in this area, thus representing an important guaranty of coherence, quality, and security for patients.[22] Indeed, as Ruth Deech, who from 1994 to 2002 chaired the British Human Fertilization and Embryology Authority (HFEA)—the British equivalent of the French ABM[23]—stated in a special recent issue of the *Hastings Center Report* fully devoted to ART and entitled "Just Reproduction: Reimagining Autonomy in Reproductive Medicine,"[24] such systematic national supervision favors the homogeneity and quality of care and is a guarantee for the citizens, especially in terms of healthcare security as well as for researchers and practitioners: "British regulation [of ART activities] has reassured the public that these areas of science and medicine are being responsibly overseen and has reduced commercialism.... It has caused everyone involved to think, justify and monitor his or her research and practice, knowing that they will be visible to the HFEA.... It has enabled progress to be made in tandem with public acceptance and has created a safe zone for the practitioners and the researchers."[25]

Ethical Limits of the Model

Although the French model of access to ART was considered to have a strong ethical foundation, symptoms of a notable mismatch between the regulations and some important societal values became increasingly obvious every day. Here, we detail some significant ethical limits of this model.

A first limitation, which should significantly change with the 2020 law, was linked to the number of those "left out" of the system, which increased year after year due to societal evolution and diversification of the ways to create families. The concerned people all claimed that the model was unfair and asked for a better consideration of their rights to be respected with regard to their reproductive autonomy and private life choices. Furthermore, they felt discriminated in their rights to have access to the same healthcare services as everyone else. They also contested the fact that the costs for accessing healthcare were conditioned by considerations of sex, sexual orientation, or form of relationship status. Indeed, on all these different points, they were increasingly supported by society at large, as confirmed by national surveys. According to one of the latest such surveys, conducted in December 2017, 60% of French people were in favor of opening access to sperm donation and ART to lesbian couples, compared to 24% in 1990; 57% were in favor of opening it to single women and 64% were ready to support legalization of gestational surrogacy.[26] This evolution can most likely be explained by a national trend toward according more importance to respect for personal autonomy. This shift has extended to opening oocyte vitrification for elective fertility preservation: with the recent law, the procedure becomes available to women for reason of age, which today represents in other developed countries the major part of such requests. So far, in France, only women facing the threat of infertility due to a medical condition or a medical treatment were allowed to preserve their eggs. Thus, even if the 2020 law does not raise all the limits of access to ART,[27] the trend is in favor of a much greater respect for reproductive autonomy.

Another important ethical limit of the French model that has become evident over the years is the barrier to scientific and technological progress resulting from ART restrictions. Researchers in France regularly denounce the scientific delay they experience compared to their foreigner colleagues due to the fact that they cannot test any innovative research approach or propose a new reproductive technology to become available for daily clinical practice without ABM authorization and/or the law being reviewed. A good example of the negative impact of the model on the professional performance of French teams working in reproductive technologies is seen in the techniques of egg-freezing and egg-reutilization after freezing. Because access to such techniques was limited, their performance could not be as successful as in countries that regularly practice them. Thus, if it is true that, on the one hand, regulation favors, as Ruth Deech states, the security of care because teams have to work under scrutiny and transparency, on the other hand, too strict rules may have negative consequences in terms of ART success rates and quality of care, which is pejorative from an ethical point of view, a point Deech also recognizes: "The downsides of regulation are that it can be slow and expensive and a barrier to progress."[28]

A last example of significant ethical concern for the French model of ART access is linked to the increasing fragility of its founding set of values, as illustrated by the 2020 law. In opening ART access to lesbian couples and single women, it undermines the indisputable barrier between infertility for medical or nonmedical reasons that regulated ART access until now. This first breach might open the road for others. For example, the recent law did not change the regulation about age, which is still considered as a regulating nonmedical criterion of access to ART: in France, women's access to ART is not permitted above the age of 43, considered the mean age of "natural" infertility. But some women have contested this interdiction. They contend that the biological clock is a strong limit for them that could be technically circumvented by medicine, and because it is not the same for men, the regulation engenders important inequalities between males and females.

Furthermore, the noncommodification principle, another important principle on which the model was constituted, has also become somewhat weakened. Not so much as far as donors are concerned—the French population remains very strongly attached to the principle of anonymity and gratuity of body part donations and the 2020 law maintains it[29]—but with respect to the recipients, or rather the children conceived with donors gametes. Because many of them requested access to their genetic identity or at least claimed to have the choice to do so, the regulation is in the process of being changed to authorize access if the donor gave their agreement at the time of donation.[30]

Finally, one can wonder if the third founding principle of access to ART, which associates the authorization of access to ART to the reimbursement of the costs of using ART, will resist important extensions of access authorized by the new law. As French society remains very attached to the egalitarian system supported by universal health coverage, the new changes were voted together with the conservation of all conditions that guarantee reproductive justice. Indeed, there were strong counterarguments to deciding to open access to ART for nonmedical reasons without reimbursing the costs of its use in these circumstances. It would have been contrary to the principle of full collective and financial solidarity vis-à-vis any medical/therapeutic need of any patient, which is a cornerstone of the French healthcare system, unless one decided not to pay for ART for anyone, even those with pathological infertility. This would then introduce inequality of access to healthcare somewhere else in the system: between patients suffering from infertility and patients suffering from other diseases. Furthermore, such a move would remove regulation from the state's domain and expose requesters to what Elizabeth Reis and Samuel Reis-Dennis call "the moral risks of commercialized fertility."[31] Conversely, opening access to ART for nonmedical reasons while paying for everybody who requests this treatment risks financial difficulties for the public health budget. Funding is not without limits, and providing additional services may extend access times to rare resources (anonymous sperm, ART specialists), or be done at the expense of other health expenditures. How should the priorities be made, and who should make them? Is the new model realistic? The issue is an authentic ethical one, and debate continues.

In conclusion, our opinion is that the French model of access to ART faces profound contradictions that are hard to deal with and that the 2020 law does not completely resolve. It is not evident how it is possible to find a better way to improve reproductive autonomy while simultaneously preserving a high degree of reproductive justice, as the legislation tries to achieve. Some concrete tensions in access or new claims for more respect for private choices might quickly emerge. Conversely, the American model of access to ART is also controversial, but for opposite reasons. This was the key topic of Louise King et al.'s introduction to the special issue of the *Hasting Center Report* published in 2017, "Autonomy in Tension: Reproduction, Technology, and Justice." The authors wrote: "Respect for autonomy is a central value in reproductive ethics, but it can be a challenge to fulfill and is sometimes an outright puzzle to understand. . . . Add a commitment to justice to the mix, and the challenge can become more complex still. Is it unfair for insurance policies to exclude from coverage the costs of giving fertility to those who lack it or restoring fertility in those who have lost it? What does 'just reproduction' look like in the face of multifarious understandings of both justice and autonomy and in light of increasingly complex and costly reproductive technologies?"[32] Indeed, if each model is illustrative of its referent healthcare system, which is itself a product of history and culture, each one has its own strengths and limits and has to struggle to find a satisfying balance, ethically speaking, between reproductive autonomy and reproductive justice.

References

1. The bioethics law has been under parliamentary discussion since 2019; it opens access to sperm insemination for lesbian couples and single women but maintains the interdiction of surrogacy.

2. On the concept of "just reproduction," see the special recent issue of the *Hastings Center Report*. The future of reproductive autonomy: Just reproduction: Reimagining autonomy in reproductive medicine. *Hasting Cent Rep*. 2017;47(6):S6–S11. In the first paper of this special issue, untitled "Autonomy in Tension: Reproduction, Technology, and Justice," Louise P. King and Rachel L. Zacharias wrote "Respect for autonomy is a central value in reproductive ethics, but it can be a challenge to fulfill. . . . Add a commitment to justice to the mix, and the challenge can become more complex still. Is it unfair for insurance policies to exclude from coverage the costs of giving fertility to those who lack it or restoring fertility in those who have lost it? What does "just reproduction" look like in the face of multifarious understandings of both justice and autonomy and in light of increasingly complex and costly reproductive technologies?"

3. Information report of the task force on the revision of the bioethics laws, 2010. By Claeys A (president) and Leonetti J (reporter), French National Assembly, doc. no. 2235, p. 9, p. 228 and p. 415.

4. This clarification was added in response to political and social controversies that followed several cases brought before the courts in which widowed wives requested the restoration of gametes that were frozen before the deaths of their husbands or the implantation of cryopreserved embryos in order to carry out their parental projects. This restriction was maintained in the new law project.

5. Théry I. *Des humains comme les autres, Bioéthique, anonymat et genre du don*. Paris: Editions de l'EHESS; 2010: 207.

6. In particular the Lejeune Foundation, an organization whose power to act is reinforced by the weekly online press review *Généthique*, the only French-language bioethics review of its kind.

7. See the order of the Ministry of the Health and Solidarity of June 30, 2017, concerning "Rules of Good Clinical and Laboratory Practice of Medically Assisted Procreation," II. 2.

8. With the exception of certain biological procedures that fall under the responsibility of the couple. See subchapter 9–2 of chapter 9 of book II of the common classification of medical procedures.

9. The woman, for example, must not be older than 43 years. For artificial insemination, coverage is limited to six donations (one per cycle) and, for IVF, to four attempts (oocyte collection until the embryos are transferred in utero). It should also be noted that coverage by Social Security does not place an age limit on men.

10. Article L. 2162-5 CSP: 5 years' imprisonment and a 75,000 euros fine.

11. "Nous, médecins, avons aidé des couples homosexuels à avoir un enfant même si la loi l'interdit," http://abonnes.lemonde.fr/idees/article/2016/03/17/pour-la-creation-d-un-veritable-plan-contre-l-infertilite_4884871_3232.html; Thery I, Leroyer A-M. *Filiation, origines, parentalités, Le droit face aux nouvelles valeurs de responsabilité*

générationnelle. Report submitted to the Delegate Minister for the Family, O. Jacob, Paris; 2014: chap. 7.

12. The High Council on Gender Equality, Contribution to the debate on access to ART, notice no. 2015-07-01-SAN adopted on May 26, 2015, http://haut-conseil-egalite. gouv.fr/IMG/pdf/hce_avis_no2015-07-01-san-17.pdf; Human Rights Defender, notice no. 15–18, July 3, 2015, http://www.defenseurdesdroits.fr/sites/default/files/ atoms/files/ddd_avis_20150703_15-18.pdf; the French National Consultative Ethics Committee, Report, June 15, 2017, http://www.ccne-ethique.fr/fr/publications/avis-du-ccne-du-15-juin-2017-sur-les-demandes-societales-de-recours-lassistance#. WZFmz4ppzql. This now must be debated in Parliament and voted on, which could be a long drawn-out process.

13. In traditional surrogacy, the surrogate provides her egg, which is fertilized with the intended father's sperm: conversely, in gestational surrogacy, another woman, either the intentional mother or an egg donor, provides the egg.

14. The civil penalties outlined in article 16-7 C. civ. (on the invalidity of surrogacy contracts) were accompanied by criminal penalties (art. L. 227-12 and 227-13 of the Penal Code) for any intermediaries involved, in addition to the intended parents and the woman who carried and gave birth to the child. So far, there have been very few convictions (Senate report, p. 56).

15. Milon A, pres., Richemont H, ed., *Information Report from the Taskforce on Maternal Surrogacy*, 2008, Doc. Sénat, 2007–2008, no. 421.

16. Gross M. *In Choosing gay parenting*, p. 15 *Eres*, 2012. https://journals.openedition. org/lectures/7793

17. ECHR. June 16, 2014, *Mennesson v. France* and *Labassée v. France*.

18. Law no. 94-653 amends the French Civil Code and Law no. 94-654 amends the Code of Public Health.

19. These rules were amended twice, on August 6, 2004, and July 7, 2011.

20. Article 16-6: " No remuneration may be allowed to a person who consents to experimentation on his person, to the removal of elements from his body, or the collection of products thereof." Article 16-8: "No information enabling the identification of both the person who donates an element or a product of his/her body and the person who receives it may be divulged."

21. In France, the official health agency in charge of the regulation and control of ART is the Agence de la biomédecine.

22. Articles L.1418-1 to L. 1418-8 of the CSP.

23. When it comes to ART and surrogacy, the United Kingdom is obviously an "open state" compared to France: any person, whether single, married, or unmarried and living with a partner can have access to ART; surrogacy is allowed under certain conditions which are currently in review for future amendment. Nevertheless, the Human Fertilisation and Embryology Authority was set up by the legislation as the UK's independent regulator of fertility treatment and research using human embryos, https://www.hfea.gov.uk/about-us/.

24. Just reproduction: Reimagining autonomy in reproductive medicine: Special report. *Hastings Cent Rep.* 2017;47(6). doi:10.1002/hast.797.

25. Deech R. Reproductive autonomy and regulation: Coexistence in action. *Hastings Cent Rep*. 2017;47(6):S58.
26. See the results of an opinion poll, "Les Français et la bioéthique." 2018 Jan 3, https://www.la-croix.com.
27. No changes about access to surrogacy, for example.
28. Deech, Reproductive autonomy and regulation.
29. Ibid.
30. Ibid.
31. Reis E, Reis-Dennis S. Freezing eggs and creating patients: Moral risks of commercialized fertility. *Hastings Cent Rep*. 2017;47(6):S41–S45, doi:10:1002/hst.794.
32. King LP, Zacharias RL, Johnston J. Autonomy in tension: Reproduction, technology, and justice. *Hastings Cent Rep*. 2017;47(6):S41–S45, doi:10:1002/hst.788.

SECTION III
OBSTETRIC ETHICS
Managing Pregnancy and Delivery

Overview

Obstetric Ethics

Julie Chor MD, MPH and Katie Watson JD

At its core, the field of obstetric ethics revolves around the maternal–fetal dyad and how patients, providers, society, and the law conceptualize and engage with this unique biological configuration. Gestating and delivering a baby is ordinary, common, and necessary to the survival of the human species. It also offers a mind-boggling challenge to concepts of boundary and identity: an entity that could become a person is growing inside the body of another person. So is a pregnant person one person? Two people? A new type of person who defies binary categorizations? Who gets to answer this question? And, practically speaking, what does the answer to that question change?

Whether or when obstetricians should consider a person's embryo or fetus as their second patient is often presented as the central question in obstetric ethics. When a pregnant patient directs you to think of their embryo or fetus as your second patient, whether you conceptualize it as equivalent to a second person or as an important part of their body they have directed you to treat may not change your actions in everyday practice, but it matters in a crisis. Performing a life- or health-threatening procedure to save a body part a patient can live without usually violates the principle of nonmaleficence, but this "second patient" designation tips the scales to beneficence, allowing clinicians to make recommendations and follow consents for interventions with significant risk and no physical benefit to the patient when the well-being of a "second patient" is at stake.

However, caring for pregnant people readily demonstrates that whether they and their families consider their embryo or fetus to be a patient may fluctuate throughout the course of a pregnancy in response to personal and medical circumstances and may vary according to what decisions must be made. Therefore, even an approach that defers to patient designation of fetal status should not be understood as a permanent on-or-off switch. The simplicity of a bright line after which the interests and rights attributed to patients are granted to a fetus might appeal to providers and policymakers looking for clear external definitions. However, any medical decision-making that relies on whether or not *providers* or strangers consider a fetus to be a patient must first center the perspectives of pregnant people regarding whether they want you to do so, and then must reckon with the consequences of conflicts between the views of patients, providers, and policymakers.

This section reflects perspectives on the maternal–fetal dyad from a range of disciplines: physicians in obstetrics and gynecology (Frank A. Chervenak and Timothy R. B. Johnson) and radiology (Stephen D. Brown), lawyers (Lynn M. Paltrow and Kayte Spector-Bagdady), sociologists (Jeanne Flavin), and medical ethicists (Katie Watson and Laurence B. McCullough). Of course, the essays in this section are not able to address all of the salient ethical questions in the area of obstetric ethics. These authors offer readers foundational approaches to caring for pregnant people and challenge readers to consider how these frameworks apply in specific clinical or situational contexts that are not directly addressed, such as caesarean section on patient request or caring for incapacitated pregnant patients.

Ethicist-lawyer Katie Watson examines the maternal–fetal dyad in a chapter that answers a common question: "If it's illegal for a pregnant person to have an abortion after viability, how can that same person be allowed to refuse medical treatment that might prevent fetal demise or harm?" In Chapter 11, "Refusing to Force Treatment: Reconciling the Law and Ethics of Post-Viability Treatment Refusals and Post-Viability Abortion Prohibitions," Watson explains why these standards are ethically and legally consistent, and she suggests using the concept of reproductive justice to change the traditional equation of choosing between a patient's autonomy and a clinician's beneficence toward her fetus. She concludes that pregnant people have an ethical obligation (but not a legal obligation) to maximize the health of fetuses they intend to deliver to the best of their individual ability to do so, clinicians have an ethical obligation to help each patient meet their obligation, and both must live with the moral distress that arises when their combined best efforts don't prevent harm.

In Chapter 12, "Professional Ethics in Obstetric Practice, Innovation, and Research," physician-ethicist Frank A. Chervenak and bioethicist Laurence B. McCullough take a different view in their model of professional ethics in obstetric care. They begin with historical background on the establishment of professionalism in medicine and the field of bioethics, then they explain why they reject what they call "the maternal-rights reductionism model" that imparts the pregnant person with an absolute right to make controlling decisions over their body and "the fetal-rights reductionism model" that endows a fetus with an absolute right to life that overrides the right of the pregnant person. Instead, these authors argue that embryos and fetuses become patients either when a pregnant person decides to continue a pregnancy or at viability and that they have a moral status such that others are obligated to protect them based on their status as a patient. Then they apply their approach to three different ethical challenges in obstetric practice: nondirective counseling about induced abortion, directive counseling against home birth, and innovation and research in maternal–fetal interventions.

In Chapter 13, "Doing Harm: When Healthcare Providers Report Their Pregnant Patients to the Police and Other Authorities," sociologist Jeanne Flavin and lawyer Lynn M. Paltrow ask readers to question the practice of routinely disregarding pregnant people's personal privacy in the name of protecting their unborn fetus. They argue that many instances when members of the healthcare team have notified law enforcement of a pregnant person's actions are largely due to misinterpretation or overinterpretation of child welfare laws and policies and an expanded view of "fetal personhood" that some providers believe supersedes the rights of pregnant people, including the right to privacy. The authors argue that these actions violate the core ethical principle of nonmaleficence because they have the potential to substantially harm pregnant people and their families, and they advise clinicians how to end unjust practices, policies, and laws at the level of the individual provider and our professional organizations.

Physician Stephen D. Brown moves us to pregnant people considering fetal surgery before delivery in Chapter 14, "Prenatal Counseling for Maternal–Fetal Surgery: Potential Biases, Competing Interests, and Undue Practice Variation in the World of Fetal Care." Dr. Brown's chapter analyzes multiple sources of bias that may impact patient counseling around these decisions, from individual provider factors (age, race/ethnicity, religion, etc.), specialty perspectives (obstetric-based providers vs. pediatric-based providers), and institutional culture. Dr. Brown provides strategies of how to address potential biases and stresses the value of transparency over an attempt to achieve an unrealistic goal of value neutrality.

Finally, in Chapter 15, "Ethical Issues in Academic Global Reproductive Health," physician Timothy R. B. Johnson and lawyer-ethicist Kayte Spector-Bagdady respond to the increased interest in global reproductive health activities by examining the ethical implications of these clinical, educational, and research endeavors. The authors draw from historical examples to illustrate how global reproductive health programs have failed to consider potential ethical implications, they call attention to the limitations of applying the traditional principlist model within the context of global reproductive health, and they propose alternative ethical principles that may better suited for global work.

Discussion Questions

Chapter 11: Watson, "Refusing to Force Treatment: Reconciling the Law and Ethics of Post-Viability Treatment Refusals and Post-Viability Abortion Prohibitions"
Watson observes that no man in the United States ever faces court-ordered medical treatment, with the exception of those who are imprisoned. How much of this differential treatment is based in the biological difference of capacity for pregnancy, and how much is attributable to gender roles and gender discrimination? Watson argues that a pregnant patient has an ethical obligation to their fetus, and their clinician has an ethical obligation to the pregnant patient. Would that framing of agency change anything in your approach to treatment refusals? Watson describes two cases (that of Tabita Bricci ["Ms. Doe"] in Illinois and Jesse Mae Jefferson in Georgia) that had different legal outcomes but the same clinical outcome: after obstetricians predicted almost certain fetal death without cesarean-section both women delivered vaginally. Other cases have followed the same pattern. Does the fallibility of prenatal prognostication play any role in your analysis of the ethics of forced treatment?

Chapter 12: Chervenak and McCullough, "Professional Ethics in Obstetric Practice, Innovation, and Research"
Which of the tenets of this model do, or do not, resonate with you? Do you agree that viability by definition imparts moral status to a fetus? What is the difference between labeling a fetus a "patient" and a "person"? Is the fetus of a pregnant person who never comes to a doctor still a "patient"? What is your perspective on this model's application to practice? For example, what are the advantages of shared decision-making when advising pregnant patients who intend to pursue home birth and/or active participation in home delivery when that is what they choose, for risk reduction?

Chapter 13: Flavin and Paltrow, "Doing Harm: When Healthcare Providers Report Their Pregnant Patients to the Police and Other Authorities"
Have you ever ordered a drug test on a pregnant patient? What are the reasons that justify ordering that test, and what might be potential implications for the patient? When, if ever, do you have a responsibility to notify law enforcement of a pregnant person's actions? What justifies this action?

Chapter 14: Brown, "Prenatal Counseling for Maternal–Fetal Surgery: Potential Biases, Competing Interests, and Undue Practice Variation in the World of Fetal Care"
What factors may bias how you counsel pregnant patients? Do you aspire to provide value-neutral, unbiased advice to patients? Do you plan to discuss your own sources of bias that inform your counseling with your patients? When might you do some of both?

Chapter 15: Spector-Bagdady and Johnson, "Ethical Issues in Academic Global Reproductive Health"
How should you adapt your practice in global health settings? How are the ethical considerations for reproductive health endeavors different from global health programs in other areas of medicine? Should there be distinctions? Why or why not?

11

Refusing to Force Treatment

Reconciling the Law and Ethics of Post-Viability Treatment Refusals and Post-Viability Abortion Prohibitions

Katie Watson JD

It's a common question for trainees: "If it's illegal for a pregnant person to have an abortion after viability, how can that same person be allowed to refuse medical treatment that might prevent fetal demise or harm?"

Cases raising this question are rare because most people carrying viable fetuses will agree to practically anything their physician or midwife tells them will help their baby survive. Indeed, the drive to deliver a healthy child leads some pregnant people to go to the opposite end of the scale, embracing burdensome treatments with little evidence of benefit (e.g., long periods of bed rest) or low odds of success (e.g., experimental intrauterine surgeries).

However, before urgent moments of refusal arise it is critical for clinicians to understand why the American College of Gynecologists (ACOG) Committee on Ethics has concluded that they are ethically obligated to respect a pregnant person's refusal of recommended medical interventions,[1] and why some state courts have ruled that clinicians are legally required to defer to these refusals. To help clinicians reason through these issues, I review the legal and moral status of women, viable fetuses, and women pregnant with viable fetuses to explain why these seemingly contradictory standards— prohibitions on post-viability abortion and preservation of autonomous patient decision making throughout pregnancy and delivery—are ethically and legally consistent. I argue that the principle of justice breaks the tie that some people perceive between autonomy (of women) and beneficence (to fetuses), pushing the scales in favor of women. Reproductive justice requires a model of investment in which society invests in women before, during, and after pregnancy versus a model in which society exclusively requires women to do for others, and I argue that this justice analysis holds true in moments of refusal as well.

Ethical and legal support for treatment refusals does not mean that an obstetrician confronted with such a refusal should—or ethically can—cry "patient autonomy" and give up. Instead, in the second part of this chapter, I offer ethically sound steps that obstetricians confronted with refusals should take to maximize care, and I consider the moral distress these unusual cases invariably invoke.

The Legal and Moral Status of Women

Discussion of the legal and moral status of embryos and fetuses is incomplete without discussion of the legal and moral personhood of the people in whom they reside. The American legal structures affirming that a woman is a full person whose political, social, economic, and personal worth is not less than a man's are relatively recent. Therefore, a brief review of the evolution of the legal status of women provides necessary context for discussion of the legal status of pregnant women. (Some people with the capacity for pregnancy do not identify as women, and people of all genders may experience unequal opportunity. I use the word "woman" in this historical discussion to highlight the fact that people identified as women have been targeted for unequal opportunity on the basis of their status as women for centuries [whether or not they were capable of pregnancy]. I also do so in the legal discussions of sex discrimination and forced medical treatment to reflect the courts' understanding of the litigants' gender.)

The US Constitution was ratified in 1790, but for most women of African descent in the United States, legal status as free people did not come until 1865, when slavery was abolished through the Thirteenth Amendment. Being legally recognized as free was a pivotal step, but, of course, it did not necessarily make this status a social reality.

The legal status of married women of every race was comparable to that of children before 1840. Before marriage they were subsumed in their father's' legal identity, and after marriage they had no legal existence separate from their husband. Married women could not legally own property (even when it was inherited), control their own earnings, or sign contracts. Beginning in 1840, Married Women's Property Acts gradually changed this on a state-by-state basis, but it took more than 50 years. For example, in 1872, the US

Supreme Court affirmed Illinois's refusal to give Mrs. Myra Bradwell a license to practice law despite its concession that she was qualified because lawyers must be able to enter contracts with clients, and Mrs. Bradwell's status as a married woman meant Illinois law prohibited her from doing so. Three US Supreme Court Justices joined a concurring opinion affirming this outcome, adding that women belonged in "the domestic sphere" and "the idea of a woman adopting a distinct and independent career from that of her husband" is "repugnant" to the "family institution."[2] Almost a century after Mrs. Bradwell was prohibited from being licensed as an attorney, the "domestic sphere" construct enforced in *Bradwell v. Illinois* (1872) returned in *Hoyt v. Florida* (1961). An all-male jury convicted Mrs. Hoyt of murdering her husband, and, despite the fact that the US Supreme Court had found racial discrimination in jury selection to be unconstitutional, the Court rejected Mrs. Hoyt's claim that sex discrimination in jury selection was unconstitutional. Instead, in a unanimous opinion, the Court ruled that Florida could constitutionally "conclude that a woman should be relieved from the civic duty of jury service unless she herself determines that such service is consistent with her own special responsibilities," because "woman is still regarded as the center of home and family life."[3] The Court did not reverse its position until 1975, when it held that states must include women on juries in *Taylor v. Louisiana.*

The political personhood of adult women wasn't acknowledged nationwide until 130 years after the ratification of the Constitution. The 19th Amendment, which prohibits federal and state governments from denying women the vote, was passed in 1920.

The economic personhood of women was recognized in 1963, when the practice of paying lower wages on the basis of sex was prohibited by the Equal Pay Act, and in 1964, when the practice of employment discrimination on the basis of sex was prohibited by Title VII of the Civil Rights Act. In 1974, the last vestiges of the economic restrictions that led to the Married Women's Property Acts in the 1800s were addressed in the Equal Credit Opportunity Act, which required banks to allow married and single women to apply for credit cards and loans in their own name based on their individual credit history. In 1972, Title IX of the Education Amendments recognized women's intellectual potential and educational ambitions by prohibiting the practice of gender discrimination in publicly funded education.

The 1965, 1972, and 1973 Supreme Court cases establishing women's constitutionally protected right to use contraception and abortion are discussed in detail in Chapter 6 in this volume (David A. Strauss, "Contraception and Abortion in the United States: A Brief Legal History"). For purposes of this review, their significance is that, in the late 20th century, the practice of denying US women the ability to use medical technology that gave them the ability to reliably do what men have been able to do since our species began—to have sex without having a baby afterward—was found to violate their constitutional rights. These cases (*Eisenstadt v. Baird* in 1965, giving married people the right to use contraception; *Griswold v. Connecticut* in 1972, giving single people the right to use contraception; and *Roe v. Wade* in 1973, giving all women the right to abortion) gave women a legal right to have sex for pleasure instead of just for procreation and a right to either set a life course separate from a biological or social identity as a mother or to prioritize and integrate their multiple identities as they see fit.

Federal laws against pregnancy discrimination emerged around the same time. The practice of expelling girls and women from school because they had become pregnant was prohibited in 1972 by Title IX of the Education Amendments. However, it was legal to fire employees for being pregnant until 1978, when the Pregnancy Discrimination Act amended Title VII to establish that "The terms 'because of sex' or 'on the basis of sex' include, but are not limited to, because of or on the basis of pregnancy, childbirth, or related medical conditions." In 1993, the Family Medical Leave Act (FMLA) required some employers to give their employees up to 12 weeks of unpaid, job-protected leave. (This statute protects people working for covered companies from having to choose between postpartum leave and continued employment, but because in most states there is no legal requirement for *paid* maternity leave, some people who are eligible for FMLA leave may still need to return to work quickly.) Accommodations that allow breastfeeding mothers to leave the home to participate in school, work, or public spaces while nursing or pumping remain variable.

An analysis of "the moral status of men" would seem nonsensical ("High? Baseline? Um, people?") because it is uncontested. Yet because legislators often codify moral codes into law, something important about the moral status of women is revealed by the history of their legal status. Women's moral status has been contested, and women's full personhood has only recently received wide recognition in the United States. The laws just described are about the control of women's bodies and whether and how those bodies can be in public spaces. Women's capacity to become pregnant, and an assumption that their only (or most important) role in life is to be mothers and wives living primarily or exclusively in "the domestic sphere," has been the source of legalized discrimination against women for centuries. As a result, the moment in which a woman in a contemporary hospital asserts bodily control and decision-making authority is both a unique interaction occurring between the individuals in that room and a power contest that can be seen as a part of this flow of history.

No American man ever faces court-ordered medical treatment in the United States unless he is in prison. Biology is certainly a factor in that gender disparity, but a complete explanation for that differential treatment is likely more complex.

The Legal and Moral Status of Viable Fetuses in Utero

In *Roe v. Wade* (1973), the Supreme Court held that states may ban abortion after fetal viability except when a woman's pregnancy threatens her life or health. (*Roe* did not require states to ban post-viability abortion, but most have passed laws doing so.) *Roe*'s viability line has led to a common misunderstanding: that *Roe* held a fetus is "a person" at viability. That is incorrect, and understanding what the *Roe* Court actually ruled is important because of the way abortion politics can (consciously or unconsciously) influence our response to treatment refusals.

Legally, the *Roe* Court concluded that the use of the word "person" in the Constitution only applies after birth. The text of the Constitution itself uses the word "person" 16 times. The Constitution does not define the term, but the *Roe* Court found no outside evidence that the Framers intended to include fetuses in the category of the "people" whose rights were being defined, and simple examination of the text revealed to them that no use of the word "person" in the Constitution "has any possible pre-natal application."[4] Postcolonial history played a role in the Court's textual analysis as well: "[T]his, together with our observation, supra, that throughout the major portion of the 19th century prevailing legal abortion practices were far freer than they are today, persuades us that the word 'person,' as used in the Fourteenth Amendment, does not include the unborn."[5] (A note on language: The *Roe* Court's conclusion, that the word "person" in the Constitution does not include "the unborn" makes it repetitive for me to add "in utero" after the term "viable fetus" in this section's heading because, legally and medically, the term "fetus" only applies in a person's uterus. [When a viable fetus is delivered, it is then called a preemie, neonate, infant, or baby.] However, my grammatical error of calling the subject of this discussion a "viable fetus *in utero*" seems a necessary corrective to a larger cultural error, in which fetuses are inaccurately depicted [both visually and imaginatively] as separate from the women in whom they live. The same concern leads me to use terms like "a fetus," "fetuses," or "her fetus" rather than "the fetus." "The fetus" is an independent abstraction, rather than an embodied entity, which immediately frames our subject as an object of public concern. I think it's more productive to begin in a neutral or possessive place, then to reason one's way from there about whether the public [via their elected representatives] or physicians [via power vested in them by courts or legislatures] should or should not have a role in deciding what happens with, to, and for any particular fetus, or fetuses generally.)

Roe did not give rights to fetuses in utero at any point of development. Instead, it ruled that a state has an interest in "potential human life" that it may seek to protect through its laws. This raises some rarely articulated questions: What exactly justifies the government's interest in potential life inside a woman's body that is not a "person" under the Constitution? (A governmental interest in creating more taxpayers? More soldiers?) Given that *Roe* held that fetuses are not "persons" protected by the Constitution until delivery, why did it also hold that states may limit the freedom of someone who *is* a person protected by the Constitution (a woman) to terminate her pregnancy at any point she chooses? The *Roe* Court phrased it this way: "The pregnant woman cannot be isolated in her privacy. . . . [I]t is reasonable and appropriate for a State to decide that at some point in time another interest . . . that of potential human life, becomes significantly involved. The woman's privacy is no longer sole and any right of privacy she possesses must be measured accordingly."[6]

Yet "potential human life" exists at every point in pregnancy. Why did the *Roe* Court decide that the state's "important and legitimate interest in potential life" becomes "compelling" at viability? Pushing beyond the Court's legal reasoning on this point can help illuminate something about the moral status of viable fetuses.

The *Roe* Court only offered two sentences explaining its choice of the viability line: "This is so because the fetus then presumably has the capability of meaningful life outside the mother's womb. State regulation protective of fetal life after viability thus has both logical and biological justifications."[7] The Court repeated the *Roe* rationale for the viability line in *Planned Parenthood v. Casey* (1992), but the *Casey* Court's most significant contribution on the topic may lie in its use of the term "workable": "We must justify the lines we draw. And there is no line other than viability which is more workable."[8]

The two ethical approaches to abortion regulation that can be clearly operationalized in law are autonomy (the pregnant person decides throughout pregnancy) and what philosophers call "single-intrinsic-property theories" (no abortion after embryonic or fetal development point X). In practice, the viability line incorporates both of these approaches, deferring to autonomy until fetal lungs (and all other organs) are developed enough to permit a "realistic possibility" of existence outside the womb, at which point states may use the possibility of extrauterine survival to supersede the woman's autonomy, except when the pregnancy threatens her life or health.

Viability is unique among developmental lines because it is the only developmental line that considers a woman and her fetus in relationship to one another. All other biological developments proposed as "single intrinsic property" turning points (cardiac activity, pain capacity, organized cortical activity, etc.) focus exclusively on embryos and fetuses. The viability standard takes what could be a single-intrinsic property approach like the others and expands it beyond lung development to include all bodily systems. (For example, a fetus with working lungs but missing kidneys is not "viable.") It also refocuses the standard on the ultimate biological goal of gestation—survival outside the womb—as opposed to the development of only one organ or one capacity. These tweaks make viability the only developmental standard that does not completely erase women from the analysis, although it can be criticized for only focusing on women's biological role in gestation and excluding analysis of them as thinking people and moral agents. The other single-intrinsic property approaches to abortion bans purport to be grounded in biology, but they ignore the central biological fact that embryonic and fetal development cannot occur unless those entities are located within and sustained by a woman's body.

A second way in which one could argue that the most "workable" line is the viability standard's definition of "a realistic possibility of meaningful life outside the womb" is the way it aligns abortion care with neonatology care. The preemies that fill our neonatal intensive care units (NICUs) are legally people, so allowing states to restrict abortion at the same developmental point after which we use medical technology to try to save fetuses delivered prematurely comports with what philosophers call "coherence of attitudes," or "moral coherence." In ethics the search for consistency is called "casuistry," in law it's called "precedent," and at home it's called "fairness"—the desire to see like cases treated alike.

However, it must be argued, and not simply assumed from the fact of gestational age, that cases of post-viability abortion and premature delivery are like cases. Two things distinguish the case of a woman who is 24 weeks pregnant who asks for an abortion and a woman who is in premature labor at 24 weeks and wants doctors to "do everything." The first is fetal location: the first fetus is inside the woman's body, and the second fetus is about to be expelled outside her body, where it can be cared for by others. A second difference is patient decision-making: the person in the first case doesn't want her pregnancy to result in a child, and the person in the second case does. Obstetricians who do both abortions and premature deliveries in the gray zone (sometimes on the same shift) and obstetricians who do post-viability abortions in states in which they are not banned for reasons other than maternal life and health have concluded that following their adult patient's wishes until their fetus leaves their body and becomes a second patient is morally coherent. For them, "treating like cases alike" means respecting all adult decision-makers, whether or not they are pregnant.

The *Roe* Court's decision that a fetus isn't a legal "person" until birth, yet states can force women to continue pregnancies against their will for the last 4 months of pregnancy, is a significant intrusion on bodily integrity and liberty that's rarely analyzed. In this sense, *Roe* itself is a major compromise. As discussed earlier, there are good arguments in favor of the viability standard, and the *Roe* Court's poorly explained assertion—that at some point in gestation advancing fetal development should change the abortion right—accords with a common moral intuition that philosophers call "gradualism."[9] However, using lung development as the moment a state may stop a woman from ending an unwanted pregnancy also creates what I call the *viability paradox*: because a fetus could survive *outside* a woman's body, the law can force a woman to carry an unwanted viable fetus *inside* her body. The viability line for abortion bans fails to match its moral claim (it's when fetuses could live outside women's bodies) with its practical outcome (therefore it's when women are required to keep fetuses inside their bodies). If a fetus in utero is not a person within the meaning of the Constitution, there is a strong argument that a woman's privacy is indeed "sole" and the constitutional protection of the abortion right should continue throughout pregnancy. As a result, the burden on women who are legally compelled to carry unwanted pregnancies after viability is underappreciated.

If we agree that the moral status of viable fetuses in utero is contested, the question becomes whose determination of that moral status matters most in a conflict? Or if we conclude that there is consensus that viable fetuses in utero have some or much moral status, the question becomes whether someone other than the person in whom they live could be responsible for protecting what that second adult defines as this fetus's interests?

Women with Viable Fetuses in Their Uteruses: Legal Status

The US Supreme Court has not considered the question of post-viability treatment refusals, but (as discussed earlier) *Roe* held that state bans on post-viability abortion are permitted by the Constitution, and most states have chosen to pass these bans. So why should we conclude that the US Supreme Court would find that women must be allowed to refuse recommended medical treatment when that refusal could or will lead to the same outcome as a post-viability abortion done for reasons other than maternal life or health?

One answer lies in the difference between commission and omission. Abortion is an act of commission that interrupts nature's course, and treatment refusal is an act of omission that lets nature take its course. Abortion actively ends a pregnancy that would have continued, and treatment refusal passively allows a pregnancy that would have ended to do so.

The distinction between commission and omission has been central to the US Supreme Court's analysis of the end-of-life issues of treatment refusal and physician-assisted suicide. In *Vacco v. Quill* (1997)[10] physicians and patients argued that allowing patients to refuse life-saving medical treatment while criminalizing physician-assisted suicide (PAS) violated the Equal Protection clause of the Constitution, which requires state laws to treat "similarly situated" groups alike. The Court rejected the *Vacco* plaintiffs' claim that patients refusing life-saving treatment and patients requesting assisted suicide were similarly situated. Instead it held that the New York laws had "reaffirmed the line between 'killing' and 'letting die,' "[11] that the distinction between treatment refusals and assisted dying was both important and logical,[12] and that it followed "a longstanding and rational distinction."[13] "The distinction comports with fundamental legal principles of causation and intent. First when a patient refuses life-sustaining medical treatment, he dies from an underlying fatal disease or pathology; but if a patient ingests lethal medication prescribed by a physician, he is killed by that medication."[14] Furthermore, a physician who follows a patient's refusal intends "only to respect his patient's wishes" but a physician who assists suicide must also intend the patient's death.[15] "Similarly a patient who commits suicide with a doctor's aid necessarily has the specific intent to end his or her own life, while a patient who refuses or discontinues treatment might not. . . . The law has long used actors' intent or purpose to distinguish between two acts that may have the same result."[16]

The *Vacco* analysis applies to our question as well: permitting pregnant people to refuse unwanted post-viability medical treatment while allowing states to prohibit them from receiving a post-viability abortion for reasons other than maternal life and health follows the same distinction between commission and omission as well as the distinction between causation and intent.

Another relevant legal concept is the duty to rescue, and lack thereof. In the United States, people have a legal and ethical duty to refrain from actively harming one another, which is expressed in laws and social norms prohibiting assault. However, Americans are not assigned a legal duty to rescue one another, except in two circumstances. The first is when your action is what creates the danger the person faces. For example, if you push someone into a lake, even if your action was an accident, your rescue of that person is no longer an optional "Good Samaritan" act: it is required. This duty-to-rescue exception does not apply to pregnant women because they lack the requisite agency: when placental abruption is causing declining oxygen levels, it is inaccurate to say "she" is putting her viable fetus in danger. The source of the danger is "her body" or "nature," such that rescue makes her a Good Samaritan, but it is legally not required.

A second, more relevant, scenario that can create a duty to rescue involves "special relationships." These are relationships or roles that create a heightened duty of care, and parents and children are a classic example. If it's my child who stumbles into the lake, even though his peril is not my fault, I have a greater ethical duty (and perhaps greater threshold of risk that I'm ethically required to take) to save him than does the stranger standing next to me.[17]

However, in the United States, special relationships do not create a legal duty to rescue when it involves bodily risk or invasion. We hope parents will jump in to donate kidneys or bone marrow to save their dying children, but they are never legally required to do so. This remains true even when one could argue that the child's life-threatening health problem is the parent's (or the parent's body's) "fault," as in cases of inherited genetic conditions. However, the fact many parents rush to give their child the marrow or organ they need suggests it's an ethical obligation for those who are able to do it.

(The "special relationship" between parent and child forms the basis of pregnant women's *ethical* obligations to fetuses they intend to carry to term, which is discussed later.)

State courts that have considered the question of forced treatment of pregnant patients have not explicitly relied on the difference between commission and omission. (Many were decided before 1997, but this includes those decided after *Vacco v. Quill* as well.) Some have relied on the lack of a legal duty to rescue, which is illustrated by the paradigmatic case of *McFall v. Shimp* (1978), in which a lower court refused Robert McFall's request for a court order to force his cousin to "donate" bone marrow to save him from his aplastic anemia,[18] and 3 weeks later Mr. McFall died.[19] ("The common law has consistently held to a rule which provides that one human being is under no legal compulsion to give aid or to take action to save another human being or to rescue. . . . For our law to compel defendant to submit to an intrusion of his body would change every concept and principle upon which our society is founded. To do so would defeat the sanctity of the individual, and would impose a rule which would know no limits, and one could not imagine where the line would be drawn.") Other state courts have followed the law allowing adults to refuse any and all medical treatment, holding that pregnancy does not revoke these rights and therefore women's interests should not be "balanced" with fetal or state interests. (The ACOG Committee on Ethics reaches the same conclusion in its ethics analysis: "Pregnancy is not an exception to the principle that a decisionally capable patient has the right to refuse treatment, even treatment needed to maintain life.") In contrast, other state courts have issued orders allowing forced treatment after concluding that state laws criminalizing post-viability abortion shift a viable fetus's legal status to that of a child and/or that the compelling "state interest in life" identified in *Roe* allows the state to intervene on a viable fetus's behalf under the same child-protective rationale. Because judicial opinions from Illinois and Georgia illustrate these divergent approaches, these cases are summarized in an appendix to this chapter for those who want to learn more.

Women with Viable Fetuses in Their Uteruses: Moral Status

It is a devastating assault on a woman's humanity to treat her will and her body as inconvenient blankets that a clinician can simply push aside to reach her fetus and that is why a third party forcing medical treatment on or through a woman's body for benefit of her viable fetus is not analogous to taking temporary custody of an infant to treat it while its mother objects at the bedside. If pregnant women are only allowed to make medical "decisions" when they agree with physicians, then all their consents to high-stakes medical intervention during pregnancy are meaningless. Commandeering these decisions after refusal reveals that physicians, hospitals, and legal authorities were only giving women the moral status of "vessel" throughout pregnancy rather than the full personhood of an autonomous decision-maker.

"Obstetric violence" is a relatively new term that defines forced medical treatment during pregnancy as form of institutionalized gender-based violence.[20] The term also includes other types of provider mistreatment that women experience while giving birth, such as abuse, coercion, and disrespect. In a recent study of 2,700 US women's birth experiences, 17.3% of all women reported one or more types of mistreatment, but these rates varied by race and socioeconomic status (SES). In the category of healthcare providers threatening to withhold treatment or forcing them to accept treatment they did not want during their delivery, 3.6% of white women and 6.6% of women of color reported this experience. Divided by income, 6.5% of low SES women and 3.5% of higher SES women replied "yes" on this item.[21] Forced cesareans do not occur in a vacuum: they are an endpoint in the continuum of disrespect and coercion that too many women experience in labor and delivery.

No system is perfect; all will produce some harm. Therefore, one way to frame the ethical question is "Where should harm lie?" The question is to whom or what will harm accrue, and how much harm will be inflicted with each approach? The history of women's subjugation in general, and the history of women of color's reproductive subjugation in particular, suggests that justice lies in risking harm to a small number of fetuses, as regrettable as that is, rather than risking what history suggests will be harm to a larger number of women who will be tied down, held prisoner, or cut open against their will in the belief (but not certainty) that these measures will improve fetal health.

A woman with a viable fetus in her uterus should not be punished for her choice to leave the safety of her home to come to your hospital or clinic and to ask you to partner with her in caring for her and her fetus. Like all other patients, she should be allowed to define what medical help she wants to accept. Her capacity to create life should not be used as a reason to reduce her moral status. Instead, respect for women's power to give life means refraining from attempting to usurp their authority over when and how they use that power.

However, concluding that women with viable fetuses in their uteruses have full moral *status* as human beings does not answer the question of what moral *obligations* they do or do not have: it simply establishes that women have the kind of moral status that makes forcible bodily invasion by others immoral. Similarly, that conclusion does not answer the question of what ethical obligations clinicians have to pregnant patients who reject their recommendations. These two questions are analyzed next.

A Pregnant Woman's Ethical Obligation to a Viable Fetus She Intends to Deliver

American law's protection of bodily integrity and autonomous decision-making should prevent pregnant people from being forced to submit to recommended medical treatment. However, what is legally required is different from what is ethically required. As the judge who declined to order David Shimp to save his cousin's life by donating bone marrow commented, "Morally, this decision rests with defendant, and, in the view of the court, the refusal of defendant is morally indefensible."

I argue that a pregnant person has an ethical obligation (as opposed to an enforceable legal obligation) to prevent harm to a fetus she intends to deliver. However, the scope of this ethical duty varies between individuals and circumstances.

When a pregnant person intends to carry a viable fetus to delivery, the high likelihood it will become a person creates a version of a parent–child relationship. Therefore, an ethical duty to that viable fetus springs from an analogy to the "special relationship" between parents and children described earlier—the heightened duty of rescue I have when it's my child who stumbles into the lake. This does not mean a viable fetus is a child or that it is the same as a child. It means that it is likely to become the pregnant person's child in the future, that it is in danger in a way that impacts its future as a child, and that in a legal regime where the autonomous decision-making and bodily integrity of pregnant women is respected, the person in whom the fetus lives is the only person who can help it.

However, the scope of this ethical obligation is not infinite. It is limited by ability and reciprocity.

Ability: The boundaries of this ethical obligation encompass what each pregnant person can reasonably do within the context of their life and resources. Efforts that are ordinary for a financially secure, childless woman with a supportive partner might be extraordinary for a woman who is poor, addicted, coping with intimate partner violence, or already caring for other children. Beginning with ability shifts standard-setting from a fetal focus ("this fetus needs X, so a woman who fails to provide X is providing substandard care") to a maternal focus ("this woman is reasonably able to provide her fetus Y, so even if her fetus needs something more or different than Y, she has fulfilled her ethical obligation").

Reciprocity: Justice also requires that the pregnant person's ethical obligation to care for her fetus is proportionate to the care they have received from the world. An obligation of reciprocal care is the logical corollary of President Kennedy's famous charge, "Of those to whom much is given, much is required." So what is required of those to whom *not* much is given? Justice suggests, "not much." In a country in which we do not guarantee access to healthcare, it is unfair to demand that a marginalized woman provide a type of care for her fetus that she may or may not have ever received and to impose a duty to rescue her fetus that no one owes her. A pregnant woman who intends to deliver a child has an ethical obligation to maximize the health of her future child that is proportional to her ability to do so and proportional to the care she has received from others.

The principle of justice breaks the tie some people perceive between autonomy (of women) and beneficence (to fetuses), pushing the scales in favor of women. Reproductive justice requires a model of investment in which society invests in women before, during, and after pregnancy versus a model in which society exclusively requires her to do for others. Justice is the principle that asks of her only that which is reasonably possible in the context of her life and that asks a physician to form a supportive partnership that focuses on the pregnant patient and (when helpful) provides resources that expand what is possible for her.

Clinicians' Ethical Obligations to Pregnant People

Rather than speaking of having one patient or two patients, the ACOG Committee on Ethics wisely advises that "it is more helpful to speak of the obstetrician-gynecologist as having beneficence-based *motivations* toward the fetus of a woman who presents for obstetric care, and a beneficence-based *obligation* to the pregnant woman who is the patient."[22] However, because it is rarely in a patient's best interest to deliver a baby with an avoidable disability or to have an avoidable loss, clinicians' beneficence-based obligation to their pregnant patient can lead to fetal harm prevention. Clinicians and patients may disagree on methods, but they are typically unified in desired outcomes. Therefore, clinicians should resist the false construct of maternal–fetal conflict. (Which, as Professor Michelle Oberman observes, is actually maternal–doctor conflict.[23]) Unless fetal death or injury is her actual goal, you and your patient are on the same team. In addition, as discussed earlier, every patient has an ethical obligation to the person who may emerge from her womb in the future. Therefore, it is in her best interest to receive her healthcare team's support in meeting that obligation. You are not responsible for her fetus—she is. Your goal is to empower and enable her to do what's best for herself and her fetus and to help her make decisions she can live with.

This is why clinicians can and should use the types of persuasion described here. In addition, any moral distress you might experience after decisions are made and outcomes are experienced might be decreased by knowing you did all you reasonably could to persuade and partner with your patient toward a positive outcome.

Guidance for Ethical Action in Difficult Moments

When you are at loggerheads with a pregnant patient who is refusing your medical recommendations, respecting her autonomy is not synonymous with disengaging. Refusals that might endanger a viable fetus evoke strong emotions (the pain of fearing fetal harm, anger about patient challenges to your authority or good intentions, etc.) and that might make emotional abandonment of your patient appealing. But if you are concerned about the survival or well-being of her fetus, resist the temptation to use "following patient autonomy" as an excuse to stop caring about or advocating for your patient.

Instead of walking away (physically or emotionally) or attempting to force treatment, step back to consider your patient's motivation. Why might a pregnant patient refuse a physician's recommendation in the third trimester? There are at least three reasons and discerning your patient's reason for refusal will guide your next steps.

Reason for Refusal 1: Lack of Understanding

The patient does not understand the risks and benefits of the intervention you recommend.

High-stakes refusals must be "informed refusals." This standard is parallel to informed consent. If you think a patient does not understand the risks and/or benefits of your recommendations, you cannot yet accept her refusal.

A patient's lack of understanding could be based on knowledge barriers like low health literacy, simple misunderstanding caused by poor clinician communication, social and emotional barriers like mistrust that (in your opinion) distorts her interpretation of medical information, or distractions that make it hard for her to process the information (like physical pain or a panicked effort to summon her partner to the hospital). In these situations, your job is to reformat the information or your approach in a way that allows her to truly hear and accurately process the information you believe is critical. Who is the best person to deliver this information? In what phrasing or order is the information most likely to be understood? What physical or social circumstance is most likely to facilitate her ability to process and weigh the information? Is there someone she needs to discuss it with before she can decide?

Alternatively, sometimes a patient's lack of understanding suggests a genuine lack of capacity. If it is possible your patient might not have the *ability* to understand risks and benefits, your job is to do a thorough capacity evaluation yourself or with the help of other experts. If your patient does not have capacity, identify the appropriate surrogate decision-maker and ask him or her for informed consent or informed refusal using the substituted judgment standard—What would the patient choose if she could?—and if the surrogate does not have the necessary information about her values or priorities to do that reasoning, use the best interest standard. In this situation, you should also seek your patient's assent to every intervention or decision.

Reason for Refusal 2: Lack of Ability to Follow Recommendations

The patient understands and agrees with your assessment of risks and benefits, but other factors or values lead her to refuse the intervention you recommend.

In some cases a patient understands and agrees with her clinician's assessment of medical risks and benefits, and her refusal is driven by her assessment of nonmedical risks and benefits.

One category of these cases is driven by competing values. Religious examples of a value conflict include the women in the Illinois and Georgia cases discussed in the appendix—Jessie Mae Jefferson and Tabita Bricci (aka "Ms. Doe's") refused c-section and Darlene Brown refused transfusion because they prioritized the spiritual risks of treatment over its medical benefits. A secular example of a value conflict might be an assault survivor for whom a value like "staying in control of my body" weighs more than it does for women who have not endured assault.

A second category of these cases is driven by competing circumstances. For example, a pregnant woman with preeclampsia may understand and agree with your assessment of the medical benefits of staying in the hospital, yet she intends to leave against medical advice because she has no one else who can care for her young children at home or because she can't afford the hospital bills she fears staying would incur.

When nonmedical values or circumstances are outweighing the medical value of the recommendation, try to change the value scale. Can you give the assault survivor power or support that tips the scale enough to allow her to prefer the recommended medical intervention? Can you accurately determine and/or confidently waive charges? Can your hospital make an exception to its rule against children sleeping in patient rooms overnight or dispatch a nanny service funded by donors? Any clinician or institution that purports to care for a pregnant woman's viable fetus must care for her and her existing children as well. Refusals based in religious beliefs are more difficult, but patient beliefs about options and outcomes should still be explored. (Are there alternate treatments that are acceptable? Would she like to hear her congregational leader's thoughts about her situation?) However, principles of religious freedom and pluralism require clinicians to support patients' religious choices.

A third category of these cases is driven by overwhelming emotions that can interfere with cognitive reasoning: intense fear of being cut open in an unexpected c-section, defensive disbelief or profound disappointment about these new medical facts, utter panic that this is all happening too fast, anxiety that this time will be just like last time's terrible experience, etc. Validate these feelings (none of them is "wrong," they are part of your patient's authentic human reaction to bad news) and see if you can collaborate in reducing their intensity to a level at which they are no longer barriers to the thought processes she would otherwise use in these circumstances. If time does not allow for this level of engagement, or if it is not successful, the question is whether you can help her make medical decisions she can live with during this moment of intense emotion.

Reason for Refusal 3: Disagreement

The patient understands what you have said about the risks and benefits of the intervention you recommend, but she disagrees with your recommendation.

Imagine a patient who has had three previous c-sections. You recommend a scheduled c-section, but she insists on attempting vaginal birth after cesarean (VBAC). What can you do?

It is never ethical to coerce or manipulate a patient into following recommendations. Freedom from coercion and manipulation is one of the three pillars of informed consent (alongside discussion of pertinent information and patient agreement),[24] and the use of coercion or manipulation destroys the ethical and legal validity of informed consent. However, it is important to distinguish these negative tactics from persuasion. Because having a child with avoidable injury or demise is rarely in a person's best interest, persuasion is what clinicians should attempt when a patient's refusal is fueled by disagreement.

Coercion is a form of overpowering that "involves threats that are intended to control patients' behavior and that patients find irresistible."[25] ("I won't give you an epidural unless you do X.") Manipulation is a form of trickery that involves misrepresentation of information concerning the nature of the patient's condition or the nature of the proposed intervention.[26] ("Your baby will die if we don't do Y" when really the odds of death are less than 100%; requiring bed rest without disclosing the lack of evidence supporting the recommendation, etc.) Clinicians should confirm the most recent evidence supporting their recommendations to avoid accidental manipulation through citation of inaccurate odds.

The ACOG Committee on Ethics discourages clinicians "in the strongest possible terms from the use of duress, manipulation, coercion, physical force, or threats, *including threats to involve the courts or child protective services,* to motivate women toward a specific clinical decision"[27] (emphasis added). For example, in 2010, in Virginia, Michelle Mitchell agreed to a c-section after her provider threatened to get a court order requiring it because they suspected she was delivering a large fetus.[28] In 2014, Jennifer Goodall received a comparable threat by letter: after she refused a scheduled c-section, her hospital wrote that its physicians would do the surgery with or without her consent if they deemed it clinically necessary. Ms. Goodall had three previous cesarean deliveries and said she would consent to surgery if there was a problem during labor but she wanted to try for a vaginal delivery. The hospital's threat led her to go to another hospital for her delivery, where she consented to a cesarean section when it appeared medically necessary.[29]

In contrast, persuasion "is an attempt to convince the patient to act in a certain way by providing rational argument and accurate data. Persuasion respects patient autonomy and, indeed, enhances it by improving the patient's understanding of the situation."[30] The ACOG Committee on Ethics uses the term "directive counseling," in which the clinician "plays an active role in the patient's decision making by offering advice, guidance, recommendations, or some combination thereof." Clinicians should describe the information that is motivating their recommendation in a way that is persuasive rather than manipulative—for example, sharing the clinician's personal experience witnessing anoxic injuries and their long-term outcomes in addition to data on the issue might be appropriately persuasive.

When a patient's disagreement with medical recommendations threatens a high likelihood of significant harm to her fetus, clinicians are ethically obligated to attempt to persuade her to choose otherwise, and they are ethically prohibited from using coercion or manipulation to accomplish this goal.

Reason for Refusal 4: A Patient's Lack of Concern or Empathy for Her Fetus

Do some people who have carried a pregnancy past viability actively wish their fetus harm? It is easy to imagine how a clinician under stress could jump to this disparaging conclusion: "Refusing my recommendation could cause her fetus harm, so that must be what she wants," or "She's selfish—she's only looking out for herself, and not thinking of her fetus at all."

However, presuming that your patient's thought-process is grounded in good will and that she is operating at the top of her ability to take action is likely to be more accurate, and, at a practical level, partnering with your patient as someone whom you presume shares your positive desires for her fetus is more likely to be effective.

When Patients Refuse Your Recommendations:
Identifying and Addressing Moral Distress

It is awful to contemplate the possibility that a near-term fetus could suffer preventable death or injury, and the reality of being in the room with a still-born or injured baby who might have been rescued if you had been permitted to use your medical knowledge and skills the way you wanted to could be devastating. As the ACOG Committee on Ethics notes, moral distress can occur when the clinician's ethical and professional obligation to safeguard the pregnant woman's autonomy conflicts with their "ethical desire to optimize the health of the fetus."[31]

Moral distress is "[t]he experience of being seriously compromised as a moral agent in practicing in accordance with accepted professional values and standards."[32] Ethicist Denise Dudzinski underscores that "moral distress ... is not always a sign of an ethical problem, but can signal the clinician's deep sense of moral responsibility."[33] Moral distress occurs when a clinician perceives an obstacle to acting on a deeply held personal belief or their understanding of their professional obligations. For example, imagine that ethical and legal confidentiality obligations prevent a clinician from disclosing a patient's HIV-positive status to their at-risk spouse, who is also that clinician's patient. In cases of moral distress, a clinician feels a heightened moral responsibility (i.e., "I'm the only one who can help this at-risk person"), and the clinician's distress is directly related to the well-being of a patient versus a self-centered experience ("the spouse is my patient and they are at risk of harm" versus "I am harmed or disgusted or disturbed by my HIV-positive patient's secrecy"). Moral distress is often accompanied by a perception of powerlessness (in the face of legal or ethical requirements, as well as structural barriers like patient poverty) and blame often underlies it (the sense that harm can and should be prevented).

Recognizing and naming moral distress is the first step to countering its corrosive effects. If your prediction of fetal harm turned out to be correct, remember that the outcome was not certain at the time your patient made her decision, and it could have gone the other way. (For example, a review of 21 court-ordered interventions in pregnancy published in 1987 found that in almost one-third of the cases, the medical judgment was shown to be incorrect in retrospect.[34]) Remember that while you are affected by this experience and outcome, the reason your patient was the decision-maker is because she is the one who has to live with it in a practical, intimate, daily way. Understand that almost any action you take in cases like these can challenge your identity: "allowing" fetal harm could challenge one's self-image as a caring, effective medical professional, and being the perpetrator of a form of medical rape could challenge your self-image, too. Consider the population perspective and focus on the positive ways your support for patient decision-making affects the access and dignity of all pregnant people, rather than focusing on the negative outcome of a particular case. There is no "remedy" for moral distress, but actively processing it could be the balm that helps clinicians be ready for the next difficult case.

Conclusion

Cases in which patients refuse potentially life-saving treatment for their fetuses are unusual, and they are important. They can have a dramatic impact on the lives of the patient, staff, and sometimes the fetus involved in each case, and they are analytically and symbolically important to varying visions of gender equity, birth justice, and what it means to be a caring and responsible person and clinician. Allowing reproductive justice to break any perceived "tie" between a patient's autonomy and a clinician's beneficence toward her fetus could help clinicians stay engaged with their patients, focused on the way each case is part of larger patterns and principles, and mindful of the fact that the pregnant person will live with whatever decisions are made in an intimate and lasting way.

Appendix: State Cases

Illinois: Pregnant Women Make All Their Own Medical Decisions

In re Baby Boy Doe, 260 Ill.App.3d 392 (1994)

Dr. James Meserow recommended that Ms. Doe have a c-section for placental insufficiency. Ms. Doe refused, and a three-judge panel of the Illinois Appellate Court ruled that "a woman's right to refuse invasive medical treatment, derived from her rights to privacy, bodily integrity, and religious liberty, is not diminished during pregnancy. . . . The potential impact upon the fetus is not legally relevant."

Ms. Doe was first examined when she was 35 weeks pregnant. According to the court, Ms. Doe told Dr. Meserow she would not consent to either the c-section or induction he recommended for placental insufficiency "because of her personal religious beliefs. . . . Instead, given her abiding faith in God's healing powers, she chose to await natural childbirth." Two weeks later, Dr. Meserow concluded the condition of her fetus had worsened, and he and the hospital contacted the Cook County State's Attorney, which filed a petition for an order forcing Ms. Doe to undergo an immediate c-section. At an emergency hearing held in the lower court the same day the petition was filed, Dr. Meserow testified that the chances of Ms. Doe's fetus surviving "a natural labor were close to zero," that if the child were to survive natural labor he would be retarded, and that his chance of surviving c-section were close to 100%.

The lower court denied the State's motion for an injunction. The State appealed, and 3 days later the appellate court heard arguments and affirmed. The following day the Public Guardian attempted to take the case to the US Supreme Court on expedited appeal, but the Supreme Court refused to hear the case, and it refused a second time after the appellate court opinion was issued.[35] Ms. Doe transferred her care to a different hospital and doctor, and on December 29, 3 weeks after Dr. Meserow's second exam, she vaginally delivered a boy who appeared to be healthy. A few months later, the Illinois appellate court issued a written opinion explaining why it rejected the State's argument that it should grant fetuses rights and then balance those fetal rights against an adult's right to refuse medical treatment.

The Illinois Appellate Court primarily relied on federal and state precedent establishing adults' rights to bodily integrity—cases confirming that performing surgery without consent is battery. Its decision to do so was reinforced by cases in which courts refused to compel people to "donate" organs: the court reasoned that if family members can't be forced to give body parts to save the lives of living relatives, a pregnant woman can't be forced to undergo surgery to benefit her viable fetus either. It was also persuaded by another Illinois Supreme Court case, *Stallman v. Youngquist* (1988), which ruled that although a fetus that has been born alive can later sue third parties for violating its legal right to begin life with a sound mind and body, that child cannot sue its mother for the unintentional infliction of prenatal injuries. (*Stallman* stated: "[T]he law will not treat a fetus as an entity which is entirely separate from its mother," and "A woman is under no duty to guarantee the mental and physical health of her child at birth, and thus cannot be compelled to do or not do anything merely for the benefit of her unborn Child.") Finally, the court rejected the state's argument that *Roe v. Wade* (1973) implies that viable fetuses have rights. "The fact that the state may prohibit post-viability pregnancy terminations does not translate into the proposition that the state may intrude upon the woman's right to remain free from unwanted physical invasion of her person when she chooses to carry her pregnancy to term."

Ms. Doe used a pseudonym when the hospital brought her to court, but later chose to reveal in newspapers that her name was named Tabita Bricci. Her husband told a reporter that "[b]ased on their reading of the Bible, they believed that a pregnancy should not be terminated before full term."[36] The Briccis switched hospitals after their first hospital took them to court. Her second obstetrician, Dr. Marilynn Fredericksen, told a reporter that her testing led her to conclude that Ms. Bricci's baby could be delivered naturally and that later during delivery she saw no indication that the baby was not receiving enough oxygen.[37] After a short natural labor Ms. Bricci vaginally delivered Callian Bricci, a 4-pound 12-ounce boy who Dr. Fredericksen reported appeared to be healthy at delivery.

In re Fetus Brown, 294 Ill.App.3d 159 (1997)

In *Doe*, the Illinois appellate court was explicit that its ruling was limited to invasive procedures like surgery and that it was offering no comment on less invasive procedures like transfusions—a situation that arose 3 years later. Ms. Brown underwent a cystoscopy to remove a urethral mass when she was 34.5 weeks pregnant, and she lost 15 times more blood than anticipated. When Dr. Robert Walsh ordered a transfusion, Ms. Brown informed the team she was a Jehovah's Witness and refused, and no blood was given. Her hemoglobin continued to drop, and 2 days later, the state filed a motion for temporary custody of Baby Doe. At a hearing held the same day, Dr. Walsh testified that without transfusion both Ms. Brown and her fetus had only a 5% chance of survival.

The State of Illinois lost the *Doe* case after urging the court to grant and balance fetal rights. In *Brown* the State took a different tack, arguing that the court should balance the *state's* interest in viable fetuses against the pregnant woman's interests. The state was successful at the trial level—in a ruling issued the same day as the hearing, the trial court concluded that blood transfusions are "minimally invasive" and it gave the hospital administrator the right to consent to any and all blood transfusions recommended by Ms. Brown's physicians. Ms. Brown was transfused with six units of packed red blood cells beginning on the night of June 28 and continuing to approximately noon on June 29. She "tried to resist the transfusion and the doctors 'yelled at and forcibly restrained, overpowered and sedated' her." On July 1, Ms. Brown delivered a healthy baby.

On July 25, Ms. Brown appealed the order allowing her transfusion, and a three-judge panel of the Illinois Appellate Court extended the *Doe* analysis of pregnant women's right to refuse surgery to every medical decision a pregnant woman makes. "In reaching this difficult conclusion, we note the mother's apparent disparate ethical and legal obligations," the court stated. "[W]hile refusal to consent to a blood transfusion for an infant would constitute neglect [citation omitted], without a determination by the Illinois legislature that a fetus is a minor for purposes of the Juvenile Court Act, we cannot separate the mother's valid treatment refusal from the potential adverse consequences to the viable fetus."

Georgia: Courts Can Order Pregnant Women to Submit to Cesarean Surgery

Jefferson v. Griffin Spalding County Hospital Authority,
274 S.E.2nd 457 (1981)

When Jessie Mae Jefferson was 39 weeks pregnant, an obstetrician diagnosed complete placenta previa. Ms. Jefferson "had diligently sought prenatal care for her child and herself, except for her refusal to consent to a caesarean section," because the Jeffersons were "of the view that the Lord has healed her body and that whatever happens to the child will be the Lord's will." She also said she would refuse transfusion. When the hospital petitioned for a court order, the examining physician testified that a vaginal birth brought a 99% chance of fetal death and a 50% chance of maternal death, and "it is virtually impossible that this condition will correct itself prior to delivery."

In *Jefferson*, the Georgia Supreme Court affirmed a trial court's order authorizing the hospital to "administer all medical procedures deemed necessary by the attending physician to preserve the life of defendant's un-born child," adopting the trial court's reasoning as its own. The trial court relied on *Roe v. Wade* (1973), noting that abortion at this point would be a criminal act. It reasoned that "the State has an interest in the life of this unborn living human being. The Court finds that the intrusion involved into the life of Jessie Mae Jefferson and her husband, John. W. Jefferson, is outweighed by the duty of the State to protect a living, unborn human being from meeting his or her death before being given the opportunity to live." It ruled that "this child is without the proper parental care and subsistence nec-essary for his or her physical life and health" and concluded "this child is a viable human being" who was entitled to the protection of the Juvenile Court Code of Georgia. The trial court granted state agencies temporary custody of "the unborn child" and gave them authority to make all decisions concerning the birth of the child. Ms. Jefferson was ordered to submit to a sonogram, and, if it indicated that the placenta was still "blocking the child's passage into this world," she was "ordered to submit to a cesarean section and related procedures considered necessary by the attending physician to sustain the life of this child." One Justice's concurring opinion explicitly states the bal-ancing the court is doing ("we weighed the right of the mother to practice her religion and to refuse surgery on herself, against her unborn child's right to live. We found in favor of her child's right to live"), and a second concurring opinion noted the difference in the free exercise of religion between freedom of belief and freedom of action.

The Jefferson court does not offer guidance for cases in which the esti-mated odds of fetal death are lower than 99%, so it's unclear if a 50% chance of demise (for example) would lead to the same result. The court also did not explicitly address the issue of enforcement, but it's important to note that its order did not allow for Ms. Jefferson's arrest: "This authority shall be effective only if defendant voluntarily seeks admission to either of plaintiff's hospitals for the emergency delivery of the child."

The second concurrence notes that Ms. Jefferson delivered vaginally. She went to the hospital for her court-ordered sonogram, and, according to a newspaper article published three days after the court order was granted, "a third ultrasound performed Friday night [one day after the emergency hearing was conducted] showed the placenta had moved—a most unusual occurrence."

Three procedural notes must accompany the interpretation of any state court opinion allowing forced treatment.

- Court orders in these circumstances typically *permit* treatment despite patient refusal, they do not *require* it. If an individual clinician believes that what a court has permitted them to do is unethical, they can (and should) decline to do it. As the ACOG Committee on Ethics advised, "[p]rinciples of medical ethics support obstetrician-gynecologists' refusal to participate in court-ordered interventions that violate their professional norms or their consciences."[38]
- Previous rulings allowing forced treatment do not require obstetricians practicing in that jurisdiction to force treatment in future cases or to seek court involvement in future cases if they think these rulings are unethical. For example, the lower courts of Georgia are required to follow *Jefferson* if and when a comparable case is brought to them, but *Jefferson* does not require Georgia physicians to override patient refusals.
- The fact that one lower court (a.k.a. trial court) granted an order does not guarantee that another lower court in a different part of the state will reach the same conclusion because a lower court's ruling is not binding on other courts outside its jurisdiction.

References

1. ACOG Committee on Ethics. "Refusal of medically recommended tx during pregnancy." Committee Opinion Number 664, June 2016 (reaffirmed 2019), https://www.acog.org/clinical/clinical-guidance/committee-opinion/articles/2016/06/refusal-of-medically-recommended-treatment-during-pregnancy
2. *Bradwell v. State of Ill.*, 83 U.S. 130 (1872).
3. *Hoyt v. Florida*, 368 U.S. 57 (1961).
4. *Roe v. Wade*, 410 U.S. 113, 157 (1973).
5. Ibid., 158.
6. Ibid., 159.
7. Ibid., 163.
8. Ibid.
9. Little MO. Abortion and the margins of personhood. *Rutgers Law J.* 2008;39:331, 341.
10. *Vacco v. Quill*, 521 U.S. 793 (1997).
11. Ibid., 806.
12. Ibid., 800–801.
13. Ibid., 808.
14. Ibid., 801.
15. Ibid., 801–2.
16. Ibid., 802–3.
17. A useful summary of "duty to rescue" law can be found in Menikoff, J. *Law and Bioethics: An Introduction.* Washington, DC: Georgetown U Press; 2001, 128–30.
18. *McFall v. Shimp*, 10 Pa. D. & C. 3d 90 (1978).
19. Fegelman A. Judges on hot seat in battles between patients, donors. *Chicago Tribune.* 1990 Jul 22, https://www.chicagotribune.com/news/ct-xpm-1990-07-22-9003010713-story.html

20. Diaz-Tello F. Invisible wounds: Obstetric violence in the United States. *Reprod Health Matters*. 2016;24(47):56–64. Kukura E. Obstetric violence. *Georgetown Law J*. 2018;106:721–801.

21. Vedam S, Stoll K, Taiwo TK, et al. The Giving Voice to Mothers study: Inequity and mistreatment during pregnancy and childbirth in the United States. *Reprod Health*. 2019;16:77–95.

22. ACOG Committee Opinion Number 664, June 2016.

23. Oberman M. Mothers and doctors' orders: Unmasking the doctor's fiduciary role in maternal-fetal conflicts. *Nw U L Rev*. 1999;94:451–501.

24. Ibid.

25. Lo B. *Resolving Ethical Dilemmas: A Guide for Clinicians*. 6th ed. Philadelphia, PA: Wolters Kluwer; 2020; chap. 3 (informed consent).

26. Ibid.

27. ACOG Committee Opinion Number 664, June 2016.

28. Kukura. Obstetric violence, 742.

29. Ibid., 741, and citations therein.

30. Kukura, Obstetric Violence.

31. ACOG Committee Opinion Number 664, June 2016.

32. Varcoe C, Pauly B, Webster G, Storch J. Moral distress: Tensions as springboards for action. *HEC Forum*. 2012;24:51–62.

33. Dudzinski DM. Navigating moral distress using the moral distress map. *J Med Ethics* 2016;42(5):321–4.

34. Kolder VEB, Gallagher J, Parsons MT. Court-ordered obstetrical interventions. *N Engl J Med* 1987;316:1192–6. *See also* Cantor JD. Court-ordered care: A complication of pregnancy to avoid. *N Engl J Med*. 2012;366(24):2237–40.

35. Terry D. Newborn settles caesarean fight a mother's way. *New York Times*. 1993 Dec 31, https://www.nytimes.com/1993/12/31/us/newborn-settles-caesarean-fight-a-mother-s-way.html; Elsasser G. High court refuses caesarean dispute. *Chicago Tribune*. 1994 Mar 1, https://www.chicagotribune.com/news/ct-xpm-1994-03-01-9403010194-story.html

36. Terry. Newborn settles caesarean fight a mother's way.

37. Roberts P. Baby born into path of legal storm. *Chicago Tribune*. 1993 Dec 31, https://www.chicagotribune.com/news/ct-xpm-1993-12-31-9312310131-story.html

38. ACOG Committee Opinion Number 664, June 2016.

12

Professional Ethics in Obstetric Practice, Innovation, and Research

Frank A. Chervenak MD, MMM and Laurence B. McCullough PhD

Introduction

Ethics is an essential and integral component of clinical practice and research in obstetrics and gynecology. This chapter provides an ethical framework based on professional ethics in obstetrics and gynecology that is clinically practical. This framework is based on the ethical principles of beneficence and respect for autonomy and the ethical concept of the fetus as a patient. The essay deploys this ethical framework to identify the obstetrician-gynecologist's professional responsibilities in three areas of both enduring and current clinical significance: counseling patients about induced abortion, counseling patients about planned home birth, and conducting clinical research in obstetrics for fetal benefit.

Ethical Framework

Medical Ethics

Medical ethics is the disciplined study of morality in medicine. Morality in medicine comprises the attitudes, judgments, and behavior of physicians, including physician leaders, and patients, as well as the values and judgments that shape health policy. The goal of medical ethics is to improve medical morality.[1,2]

The history of medical ethics dates from the ancient worlds of Greece and Asia.[3] In its millennia-long global history, medical ethics has drawn on the disciplines of moral theology and moral philosophy to address the question of what medical morality ought to be. Medical ethics based on moral theology is known as *theological* or *religious medical ethics*.[4] Moral theology has served as a source for medical ethics for millennia because one task of faith communities is to provide meaning and direction to the core events of the human life cycle: conception, birth, childhood, adolescence (a recent social invention), adulthood, aging, infirmity, life-taking illnesses, and death.[5–10] Medicine influences every one of these stages of the life cycle, making the attitudes, judgments, and behaviors of physicians and patients; the practices of healthcare organizations such as infirmaries and hospitals; and health policy of vital importance for faith communities. Medical ethics based on moral theology has a major limitation. Ethical reasoning in a specific faith community is very difficult, if not impossible, to generalize to other faith communities because faith communities do not accept a single theological and moral authority that would apply across all faiths.

Medical ethics based on moral philosophy, or *philosophical medical ethics*, draws on concepts that are taken to be transreligious as well as transcultural and transnational. Since the national Enlightenments of the eighteenth century in Britain, Europe, and North and South America, philosophical ethics became self-consciously transnational, transcultural, and transreligious.[1,2] Philosophical ethics did so by appealing to concepts, the authority of which does not depend on divinity of any kind. If one takes the view that philosophers invent concepts in specific historical circumstances, one will be skeptical about the existence of such generalized philosophical concepts. However, it is possible for concepts to spread across religions, cultures, and nations from their point of origin. The discourse of human rights, for example, was designed from its beginnings after World War II to be deliberately transreligious, transcultural, and transnational.[11] Deliberately framed as a secular discourse of philosophical ethics, the discourse of human rights has become global and provides transnational standards to which governments can be held accountable, especially for human rights violations such as genital mutilation of girls.

Philosophical medical ethics has a major limitation: irresolvable methodologic disagreement. There have been competing methods and concepts in the global history of moral philosophy dating back to the ancient worlds of Greece and Asia. In ancient China, Confucius (551–479 BCE), in *Analects*, made filial piety the paradigmatic moral relationship.[6] This concept is simple: children are allowed to question their parents' thinking, but once the father makes a decision, it is to be unquestionably obeyed. At nearly the same time in ancient Greece, Plato (c. 428–348 BCE), in *Republic*, proposed that the just state will require removal of infants from their parents to be raised in common.[12] He made this proposal to ensure that family or tribal loyalty was not an ethically relevant consideration, so that each individual should count equally in moral judgment. There is no single philosophical method that is taken to be authoritative for all of the schools in the global history of philosophy.

Professional Medical Ethics

Professional ethics was invented in the late eighteenth century to provide a philosophical, clinically and scientifically grounded account of the physician–patient relationship as a *professional relationship*. Two British physician-ethicists invented professional medical ethics: John Gregory (1724–1773) of Scotland and Thomas Percival (1740–1804) of England.[2,13] They first drew on the philosophy of medicine of Francis Bacon (1561–1626) to argue that clinical judgment and practice should be based on what Bacon called "experience," the carefully observed and recorded results of natural and controlled experiments. Bacon's goal was to minimize bias in clinical judgment and practice because the resulting uncontrolled variation of clinical practice impermissibly harms patients. This is a nascent form of evidence-based medicine that aims to replace uncontrolled variation in clinical judgment and practice with responsibly managed variation, which is the definition of quality.

Gregory and Percival then drew on Baconian "moral science," as it was then known, to argue for clinical judgment and practice based on constitutive features of human nature that direct us to the interests of others and away from self-interest, either as individuals or as groups defined by shared self-interest. On this basis they argued that physicians should not be "men of interest" (i.e., primarily motivated by protecting and promoting the individual self-interest of the physician; for example in reputation and income, or group self-interest, as in the pursuit of social and political standing of orthodox physicians or surgeons by the Royal Colleges, which functioned as self-interested merchant guilds).

The result was three commitments that define professionalism in medicine: to scientifically and clinically competent patient care based on "experience" or evidence; to the protection and promotion of the patient's health-related interests as the physician's primary concern and motivation, keeping *individual* self-interest systematically secondary; and to the protection and promotion of the patient's health-related interests as the physician's primary concern and motivation, keeping *group* self-interest systematically secondary. Put another way, medicine is a "public trust" (Percival's phrase) and not a private merchant guild. Recent statements on professionalism, such as the Physician's Charter,[14] invoke this three-commitment concept of medical professionalism without being aware of its historical origins. These commitments are not subject to the methodologic limitations of theological and philosophical medical ethics.

Bioethics

Bioethics was invented in the United States and Great Britain in the late 1960s and early 1970s. There is scholarly dispute about which country should have pride of place.[15,16] More to the point, North American bioethics defined itself as an essential and long-overdue corrective to the millennia-long practice and norm of medical paternalism: the limitation of the patient's autonomy by the decisions and behaviors of physicians undertaken for the patient's benefit. Medical paternalism is considered impermissible because the patient, and not the physician, is best situated to determine what is in the patient's health-related and other interests and because limitations on individual autonomy in circumstances in which there is no risk of serious, far-reaching, and irreversible harm to others are impermissible. The effect—if not the intent—of bioethics was to deprofessionalize medical ethics because antipaternalism questions whether physicians can meet the three commitments that define medical professionalism.[17]

Bioethics draws on many academic disciplines, including the healthcare professions, moral theology, moral philosophy, law, and the qualitative social sciences for the concepts that are deployed to address ethical challenges in clinical practice, research, education, and health policy. This results in a major limitation: there are serious, often irresolvable differences among these disciplines, and there are also deep cultural differences. For example, as noted earlier, North American bioethics strongly emphasizes respect for patient autonomy. South American bioethics applies to concepts of humanity in methods of philosophical anthropology that emphasize the social nature of human beings. European bioethics, deeply influenced by the catastrophe of World War II and the need to prevent such war from every recurring, emphasizes solidarity. Asian bioethics emphasizes Confucian moral philosophy. Such differences prevent the creation of a bioethics that is transnational, transcultural, and transreligious, making bioethics incompatible with professional medical ethics.

Professional Ethics in Obstetrics

Professional ethics in obstetrics is based on the three commitments that define professional medical ethics generally.[2,13,18] Professional ethics in obstetrics guides clinical judgment, decision-making, practice, and research on human reproduction and the clinical management of pregnancy. In the current literature of ethics in obstetrics, there are two extremes, each of which is incompatible with professional ethics in obstetrics and gynecology.

The first extreme position is fetal rights–based reductionism, which holds that the fetus has a right to life that in all cases overrides any right of the pregnant woman to control her body and therefore make controlling decisions about the disposition of her pregnancy.[2,13] This position does not originate in philosophical bioethics because the irresolvable methodologic disputes within philosophical bioethics prevent agreement that the fetus has such rights. The only alternative source is moral theological bioethics, specifically forms of Christian bioethics that hold that the fetus has rights from the moment of conception, a position that is unique to these forms of Christian bioethics. Fetal rights–based reductionism therefore has the same limitation that any form of theological or religious bioethics has: it cannot be generalized to a pluralistic profession of medicine serving pluralistic patients in highly variable cultural and national contexts. Fetal rights–based reductionism is therefore not compatible with professional ethics in obstetrics and gynecology.

The second extreme position is maternal rights–based reductionism, which holds that the rights of the pregnant woman to control her body and therefore make controlling decisions about the disposition of her pregnancy override the right to life of the fetus.[2,13] This position originates in philosophical medical ethics rather than religious or theological bioethics. This position treats the ethical principle of respect for the autonomy of the pregnant woman as the controlling ethical consideration and discounts or rejects altogether the moral status of the fetus. ("Moral status" means that an entity is such that others have a moral obligation to protect and promote its interests.)

The limitation of maternal rights–based reductionism is that there are philosophical disputes about whether the fetus' moral status is always secondary to that of the pregnant woman. Put another way, maternal rights–based reductionism makes maternal rights and the ethical obligations that they generate absolute (i.e., having no exceptions). Because this position assumes that rights originate in individual autonomy, maternal rights–based reductionism treats respect for patient autonomy as an absolute ethical principle. Maternal rights–based reductionism is therefore incompatible with professional ethics in obstetrics and gynecology.

The Moral Status of the Fetus as a Patient

Professional ethics in obstetrics and gynecology rejects these two extremes because they share the implicit assumption that the only way to understand moral status is in terms of rights. There is an alternative view that comes from the history of professional medical ethics: the moral status of being a patient. In professional medical ethics, to become a patient is simple: a human being is presented to a physician (or other healthcare professional), and there are forms of clinical management that are reliably predicted to benefit that individual clinically.[2] In the technical language of ethics, this is a beneficence-based concept. In professional medical ethics, beneficence is an ethical principle that creates the ethical obligation to identify and provide forms of clinical management that in deliberative (evidence-based, rigorous, transparent, and accountable) clinical judgment is predicted to result in net clinical benefit (a greater of clinical goods over clinical harms). Beneficence-based ethical obligations are prima facie: they should guide clinical judgment, decision-making, and practice unless it can be shown that another ethical obligation should take priority. The ethical principle of beneficence as a prima facie ethical principle must therefore always be balanced against respect for patient autonomy, another prima facie ethical principle.[2,13]

In professional ethics in obstetrics the obstetrician has beneficence-based ethical obligations to the fetus when the fetus is a patient.[2,13] There exist forms of clinical management that in deliberative clinical judgment can be predicted to benefit the fetus around the time that the fetus is viable (i.e., can exist ex utero, albeit with technological support, especially neonatal intensive care). Viability results in the fetus becoming a patient. In all cases, this means (1) that there are prima facie, not absolute, beneficence-based ethical obligations to the fetal patient and (2) these beneficence-based obligations must be balanced against prima facie beneficence-based and autonomy-based ethical obligations to the pregnant patient. Focusing only on one of these two sets of obligations while neglecting the other is not compatible with professional ethics in obstetrics and gynecology.

The fetus can also become a patient in pregnancies that the pregnant woman elects to continue to viability. This decision, which may not always be made explicitly, results in the fetus becoming a patient to whom the pregnant woman and the obstetrician have prima facie beneficence-based obligations. The obstetrician also has prima facie autonomy-based ethical obligations to the pregnant patient. In all cases, this means (1) that there are prima facie, not absolute, beneficence-based ethical obligations to the fetal patient and (2) these beneficence-based obligations must be balanced against prima facie beneficence- and autonomy-based ethical obligations to the pregnant patient. Focusing only on one of these two sets of obligations is not compatible with professional ethics in obstetrics.[2,13]

Two Current Ethical Challenges in Obstetric Practice

Counseling pregnant women about induced abortion and counseling women about planned home birth present the obstetrician with ethical challenges. The ethical framework that we have presented provides guidance based on the distinction between nondirective counseling (offering but not recommending clinical management) and directive counseling (recommending clinical management and, when ethically justified, recommending against clinical management).

Nondirective Counseling about Induced Abortion

There are four clinical circumstances in which induced abortion should be offered based on respect for the woman's autonomy.[19] When a pregnant woman expresses an interest in ending a previable pregnancy or seems hesitant about continuing a previable pregnancy, the obstetrician has an autonomy-based ethical obligation to present the alternative of induced abortion. To elicit the woman's views, it may be helpful to ask her how she feels about being pregnant. When a pregnancy is the result of rape or incest, the obstetrician should offer induced abortion. In addition, when a fetal anomaly has been diagnosed in a previable fetus, the obstetrician has an autonomy-based ethical obligation to present the alternative of induced abortion. Finally, in a higher order multiple gestation, the obstetrician has an autonomy-based ethical obligation to present the alternative of induced abortion. Some women will reject the offer. Others will accept it.[2,19] There is a beneficence-based obligation to offer induced abortion when her pregnancy creates a risk of mortality, especially when that risk cannot be reduced as pregnancy progresses.[19]

In professional obstetric ethics, a pregnant woman who accepts the offer of induced abortion, in effect, has withheld or withdrawn the moral status of her fetus(es) being a patient. In professional ethics in obstetrics, the obstetrician therefore has no beneficence-based ethical obligation to protect fetal life. The obstetrician has the autonomy-based obligation to lead a shared decision-making process with the pregnant woman. To implement this autonomy-based ethical obligation, the obstetrician should describe clinically appropriate forms of induced abortion, their risks to the pregnant woman, and that they all result in the death of the fetus. In a shared decision-making process, the obstetrician should be strictly nondirective by making no recommendations either for or against induced abortion or expressing any moral judgment of any kind about the pregnant woman's reasoning process and ultimate decision. To do otherwise is an egregious violation of autonomy-based ethical obligations.[2,19] To prevent this violation, the obstetrician should elicit the patient's values (what is important to her for her pregnancy) and support the woman in making judgments and decisions based on her values.

Some obstetricians may have moral objections to induced abortion based on sources of morality other than professional obstetric ethics (e.g., a commitment to a moral theology that prohibits induced abortion). Such moral objection does not apply to the professional responsibility to offer induced abortion, lead a shared decision-making process, and refrain without exception from making recommendations or expressing moral judgment.[20]

Obstetricians with such moral beliefs are ethically justified in explaining to the pregnant woman that their scope of practice does not include induced abortion for personal, not professional, reasons. Such obstetricians may also take the view that their personal morality is not consistent with making a direct referral to a physician who provides induced abortion. This limitation on practice does not rule out indirect referral (i.e., informing the pregnant woman about clinics that provide nondirective professional counseling and safe and effective induced abortion). This includes Planned Parenthood but excludes so-called pregnancy crisis centers that violate the professional ethical standard of nondirective counseling by not offering induced abortion or recommending against it.[2,19]

Directive Counseling about Planned Home Birth

Planned home births are increasing in the United States. Obstetricians should therefore be prepared to respond to expressions of interest in it or a request to participate from their patients, before or during pregnancy. While the absolute risks of adverse neonatal outcomes such as death, low Apgar scores, and neurologic injury and disability are very low, studies using the largest, most reliable database have consistently demonstrated increased absolute and relative risks of perinatal morbidity and mortality when compared to planned hospital birth attended by nurse midwives.[21-24] These risks can be prevented only by planned hospital birth because of the unpreventable delays of transfer from any home birth setting. The first commitment of professional obstetric ethics, to scientifically and clinically competent patient care, requires obstetric practice to meet evidence-based standards of patient safety and quality. This is beyond dispute in professional obstetric ethics. Therefore, professional integrity never includes the knowing provision of patient care that fails to meet evidence-based standards. This creates the ethical obligation to inform the woman that there is no way to reduce the risks of perinatal morbidity and mortality by modifying the home birth setting because these changes do not create the capacity to manage the unpredictable risk of a low-risk pregnancy suddenly becoming a high-risk pregnancy that requires immediate intervention available only in the hospital setting. Birthing centers attached to a hospital have the capacity to manage this risk; the home setting will never have this capacity.

It follows that the obstetrician has a beneficence-based ethical obligation to the fetal and neonatal patient never to participate in planned home birth.[21-24] The obstetrician's response to a request to attend a planned home birth should be unambiguous: the obstetrician should state that his or her attendance would be unprofessional and therefore prohibited.[21-24]

It also follows that shared decision-making about a woman's plan for home birth should not be adopted as the standard because planned home birth is not acceptable in a safety culture. Instead, counseling should be unambiguously directive. The woman should be informed about the documented increased and absolute relative risks and that these risks cannot be eliminated in planned home birth because of unpreventable delays in transportation. Based on these clinical realities, the obstetrician should recommend against planned home birth. Women who elect to proceed with planned home birth should be provided professional obstetric and newborn care to improve outcomes as much as possible. Finally, and crucially, obstetricians have the professional responsibility to identify and address those aspects of planned hospital birth that may promote interest in planned home birth by creating a strong culture of patient safety and quality, one that reduces the rate of cesarean delivery, and by creating as home-like a setting in the hospital as possible, as with a birthing center adjacent to the labor and delivery ward.[21–24]

Ethical Challenges in Obstetric Innovation and Research for Fetal Benefit

Precision of Thought and Speech: Experimentation, Innovation, and Research

Clinically sound ethical reasoning requires precision of thought and speech about the meanings of "experiment," "innovation," and "research." An obstetrician performs an experiment when he or she uses a clinical intervention, the outcome of which cannot be reliably predicted in deliberative clinical judgment. An obstetrician undertakes innovative clinical management when he or she performs an experiment for the benefit of a current, individual patient. An obstetrician undertakes clinical research when he or she performs an organized experiment to produce generalized knowledge for the benefit of future patients.[2] To avoid imprecision of thought and speech, "experimentation" should not be equated with "research" because experimentation also includes innovation.

For both maternal–fetal innovation and maternal–fetal research, shared decision-making is essential. This is because a shared decision-making approach emphasizes nondirective counseling (i.e., offering but not recommending intervention). Nondirective counseling is required in professionally responsible innovation and research because, by definition, both are forms of experimentation. When the outcome of an intervention cannot be reliably predicted in deliberative clinical judgment, making a recommendation has no evidence base and is therefore ethically not permitted.[2,20]

It is also essential that the shared decision-making process makes clear that the proposed innovation or research should not be confused with accepted clinical practice. The goal is to prevent what is known as the *therapeutic misconception*: that proposed clinical management is accepted practice and not investigational.[2]

Professionally Responsible Maternal–Fetal Innovation for Fetal Benefit

All interventions for fetal benefit are provided through the body of the pregnant woman, whether medical (medications to manage fetal arrhythmias) or surgical management of meningomyelocele. In the past, planned medical and surgical innovation was undertaken with little or no prospective review. This changed in 2008, when the Society for University Surgeons called for prospective review and approval of planned surgical innovation by a committee created for this purpose.[25] The need for such a committee results from the organizational reality that institutional review boards (IRBs) decline to review such proposed innovations because they do not fit the definition of research in the federal regulations.

In professional obstetric ethics there is an emerging standard for maternal–fetal innovation for fetal benefit: prospective review and approval of the planned innovation by a committee, sometimes known as a *fetal therapy committee*.[2] This process requires a written protocol that includes a scientific and clinical justification, an ethical justification that anticipated risks are acceptable, and the informed consent process, which should make clear that the pregnant woman is not ethically obligated to her fetus or future child to authorize the approved innovation.

The authors have proposed criteria that should be met in the design and evaluation of planned maternal–fetal innovation.

- The proposed fetal intervention is reliably expected, on the basis of previous animal studies, either to be life-saving or to prevent serious and irreversible disease, injury, or disability for the fetal patient;
- Among possible alternative designs, the intervention is designed in such a way as to involve the least risk of mortality and morbidity for the fetal patient; and

- On the basis of animal studies and analysis of theoretical risks for both the current and future pregnancies, the mortality risk of the fetal intervention to the pregnant woman is reliably expected to be low and the risk of disease, injury, or disability to the pregnant woman is reliably expected to be low or manageable.[2,26]

Professionally Responsible Maternal–Fetal Research for Fetal Benefit

The professional standard for research with human subjects, including pregnant women and fetuses, has been well-established for at least four decades: prospective review and approval of a clinical research protocol by an IRB and a documented informed consent process. It is important to note that the risk to the fetus must be minimized, which means that, from among competing study designs, the one with least risk to the fetus should be selected even if that risk is still high.[27,28] This is not the same as "minimal risk" (i.e., risk no higher than the background risk of being a fetus). The latter would be far more restrictive than the former.[28]

The authors have proposed criteria that should be met in the design and evaluation of maternal–fetal research.

- The initial case series indicates that the proposed fetal intervention is reliably expected either to be life-saving or to prevent serious and irreversible disease, injury, or disability for the fetal patient;
- Among possible alternative designs, the intervention continues to involve the least risk of morbidity and mortality to the fetal patient; and
- Research results indicate that the mortality risk to the pregnant woman is reliably expected to be low and that the risk of disease, injury, or disability to the pregnant woman, including for future pregnancies, is reliably expected to be low or manageable.[2,26]

Professionally Responsible Transition into Clinical Practice

Given the rarity of fetal anomalies for which there is support from maternal–fetal innovation, it may not be feasible to mount research with the power to test a hypothesis. The authors have proposed criteria for the professionally responsible transition into clinical practice from both innovation and research.

- The fetal intervention has a significant probability of being life-saving or preventing serious or irreversible disease, injury, or disability for the fetal patient;
- The fetal intervention involves low mortality and low or manageable risk of serious and irreversible disease, injury, or disability for the fetal patient; and
- The mortality risk to the pregnant woman is low, and the risk of disease, injury or disability is low or manageable, including for future pregnancies.[2,26]

Conclusion

Professional ethics in obstetrics and gynecology provides practical guidance to obstetrician-gynecologists about their professional responsibilities that shape their role in counseling patients about induced abortion, planned home birth, and clinical innovation and research in obstetrics for fetal benefit. The unique feature of the approach taken in this chapter is the centrality of the ethical concept of the fetus as a patient and the professional role of the ethical principles of beneficence and respect for patient autonomy.

References

1. McCullough LB, Chervenak FA. *Ethics in Obstetrics and Gynecology.* New York: Oxford University Press; 1994.
2. Chervenak FA, McCullough LB. *The Professional Responsibility Model of Perinatal Ethics.* Berlin: Walter de Gruyter; 2014.
3. Baker RB, McCullough LB, eds. *The Cambridge World History of Medical Ethics.* New York: Cambridge University Press; 2009.
4. Kurjak, A, Chervanak FA, McCullough LB, Hasanovic A, eds. *Science and Religion: Synergy not Skepticism.* New Delhi: Jaypee Brothers Medical; 2017.
5. Young KK. Medical ethics through the life cycle in Hindu India. In Baker RB, McCullough LB, eds. *The Cambridge World History of Medical Ethics.* New York: Cambridge University Press; 2009: 101–12.
6. Young KK. Medical ethics through the life cycle in Buddhist India. In Baker RB, McCullough LB, eds. *The Cambridge World History of Medical Ethics.* New York: Cambridge University Press; 2009: 113–25.

7. Nie J-B. Medical ethics through the life cycle in China. In Baker RB, McCullough LB, eds. *The Cambridge World History of Medical Ethics*. New York: Cambridge University Press; 2009: 126–31.

8. Kimura R, Sakai S. Medical ethics through the life cycle in Japan. In Baker RB, McCullough LB, eds. *The Cambridge World History of Medical Ethics*. New York: Cambridge University Press; 2009: 132–6.

9. Baker RB, McCullough LB. Medical ethics through the life cycle in Europe and the Americas. In Baker RB, McCullough LB, eds. *The Cambridge World History of Medical Ethics*. New York: Cambridge University Press; 2009: 137–42.

10. Ilkilic I. Medical ethics through the life cycle in the Islamic Middle East. In Baker RB, McCullough LB, eds. *The Cambridge World History of Medical Ethics*. New York: Cambridge University Press; 2009: 163–71.

11. McKeon R. The philosophical basis and material circumstances of the rights of man." *Ethics*. 1948;58 (1948 Apr):180–7.

12. Plato. Republic. In Cooper JM, Hutchinson DS, eds. *Plato Complete Works*. Indianapolis, IN: Hackett; 1997: 971–1223.

13. Chervenak FA, McCullough LB, Brent RL. The professional responsibility model of obstetrical ethics: Avoiding the perils of clashing rights. *Am J Obstet Gynecol*. 2011;205(4):315.e1–5.

14. Project of the ABIM Foundation, ACP-ASIM Foundation, European Federation of Internal Medicine. Medical professionalism in the new millennium: A physician charter. *Ann Intern Med*. 2002;136:243–6.

15. Jonsen AR. The discourses of bioethics in the United States. In Baker RB, McCullough LB, eds. *The Cambridge World History of Medical Ethics*. New York: Cambridge University Press; 2009: 477–85.

16. Boyd K. The discourses of bioethics in the United Kingdom. In Baker RB, McCullough LB, eds. *The Cambridge World History of Medical Ethics*. New York: Cambridge University Press; 2009: 486–9.

17. McCullough LB. Was bioethics founded on historical and conceptual mistakes about medical paternalism? *Bioethics*. 2011;25:66–74.

18. FIGO Committee for the Ethical Aspects of Human Reproduction and Women's Health. Professionalism in obstetrics and gynecologic practice. *Int J Gynaecol Obstet*. 2017;136:249–51.

19. Chervenak FA, McCullough LB. An ethically justified approach to offering, recommending, performing, and referring for induced abortion and feticide. *Am J Obstet Gynecol*. 2009;201:560.e1–6.

20. Chervenak FA, McCullough LB. The unlimited rights model of obstetric ethics threatens professionalism: A commentary. *BJOG*. 2017;124:1144–7.

21. Grünebaum A, McCullough LB, Sapra KJ, et al. Apgar score of zero at five minutes and neonatal seizures or serious neurologic dysfunction in relation to birth setting. *Am J Obstet Gynecol*. 2013;209:323.e1–323.e6.

22. Chervenak FA, McCullough LB, Grünebaum A, Arabin B, Levene MI, Brent RL. Planned home birth: A violation of the best interests of the child standard? *Pediatrics*. 2013;132:921–3.

23. Grünebaum A, McCullough LB, Brent RL, Arabin B, Levene MI, Chervenak FA. Perinatal risks of planned home birth in the United States. *Am J Obstet Gynecol*. 2015;212:350.e1–6.

24. Chervenak FA, McCullough LB, Arabin B., Brent RL. Planned home birth: The professional responsibility response. *Am J Obstet Gynecol.* 2013;208:31–8.
25. Biffl WL, Spain DA, Reitsma AM, Minter RM, et al. Society of University Surgeons Innovations Project Team. Responsible development and application of surgical innovations: A position statement of the Society of University Surgeons. *J Am Coll Surg.* 2008;206:1204–9.
26. Chervenak FA, McCullough LB. An ethically justified framework for clinical investigation to benefit pregnant and fetal patients. *Am J Bioeth.* 2011;11:39–49.
27. Protection of Human Subjects. 45 CFR 46 2009. https://www.hhs.gov/ohrp/regulations-and-policy/regulations/45-cfr-46/index.html
28. Brody BA. *The Ethics of Biomedical Research: An International Perspective.* New York: Oxford University Press; 1998.

13

Doing Harm

When Healthcare Providers Report Their Pregnant Patients to the Police and Other Authorities

Jeanne Flavin PhD and Lynn M. Paltrow JD

Introduction

In July 2017, [1] a Salt Lake City police officer arrested registered nurse Alex Wubbels after she refused to allow him to take a blood sample from a sedated patient without a warrant or the patient's consent.[2] "I'm a healthcare worker," Wubbels said. "The only job I have is to keep my patients safe." Wubbels's act of courage and patient protection made national news.[3]

Respecting patient privacy is a core value in the care for a patient. According to the American Medical Association's (AMA) ethical principles, physicians are expected "to protect patient privacy in all settings to the greatest extent possible."[4] The American Nursing Association (ANA) interprets Provision 3 of the 2015 Code of Ethics for Nurses ("The nurse promotes, advocates for, and protects the rights, health, and safety of the patient") to include "protection of the rights of privacy and confidentiality" of personal information "from or about the patient."[5]

Patient privacy encompasses several aspects including informational privacy, decisional privacy (including personal decisions based on religion and culture), physical privacy, and associational privacy (relationships with family members and other intimates). The AMA considers patient privacy in all its forms and aspects as fundamental, "an expression for patient autonomy and a prerequisite for trust."[6] According to the AMA Code of Ethics, physicians should notify the patient if a law or court order requires them to disclose confidential information and then, pursuant to that law or order, to "disclose the minimal information required." The ANA Code obliges nurses to protect patient health and safety by "acting on questionable practice," as nurse Alex Wubbels did, including not remaining silent in the face of errors or ethical violations.[7]

Medical staff who collect and wrongfully disclose information about their patients to law enforcement officials also may be sued for damages as a result of violations of well-established constitutional rights to privacy, as well as malpractice or other torts relating to breaching the physician–patient contract.[8]

There is no exception for pregnancy mentioned in any of these codes of ethics. That is because, upon becoming pregnant, a person does not have a special, lesser status with regard to medical care and expectations of patient privacy. No less than anyone else, pregnant patients should expect that their health is a private matter and that healthcare providers will respect patient confidentiality. Yet our research has found that some hospital workers have contacted police directly on their own initiative. Others have failed to offer even modest resistance to the disclosure of private patient information when law enforcement officials have requested it without a warrant, subpoena, or court order, much less challenged the request or actively opposed it. In some cases, healthcare providers have developed collaborative policies with police in which drug tests are done to collect evidence against patients. It is also common for healthcare providers to order drug tests and disclose confidential patient information to child welfare authorities even when there is no actual statutory mandate for such testing or disclosures.

These findings emerged during the course of our earlier effort to document arrests, forced medical interventions, and other deprivations of liberty of pregnant people (all of whom were identified in public records as women), including those who continued their pregnancies to term, sought or secured an abortion, or experienced a miscarriage or stillbirth between 1973 and 2005.[9] (Our original documentation found 413 cases in the 32 years between 1973 and 2005; the National Advocates of Pregnant Women [NAPW] has identified more than 800 additional cases in the 15 years since then.)

Today, in an effort to recriminalize abortion and assert patriarchal state control over people with the capacity for pregnancy, a movement to recognize separate "personhood" rights for fertilized eggs, embryos, and fetuses is under way.[10] As our study established, abortion opponents seek to establish separate rights for fertilized eggs, embryos, and fetuses by targeting pregnant women and new mothers for arrest using feticide, child endangerment, and other laws and claims of "protecting the unborn."[11] The underpinning assumption of these arrests is that a pregnant person's actions and inactions—indeed, the very state of being pregnant—constitute some sort of actual or possible harm to a child.

Rather than protecting patient privacy from outside intrusion, providers too often have been the ones gathering information from patients and disclosing it to police, prosecutors, and other authorities with the power to deprive pregnant people and new mothers of their liberty and other fundamental rights. Of the 276 cases in our earlier study in which we were able to determine how a pregnant person came to the attention of authorities, 40% involved a woman who had been reported to the police by a healthcare provider, such as a doctor, nurse, or hospital social worker. The pattern was even more pronounced for black patients and other patients of color. In another 17% of the cases, medical providers reported a woman to child welfare authorities, who then reported her to law enforcement.

We concluded that

> Although it is often presumed that medical information is confidential and rigorously protected by constitutional and statutory privacy protections as well as principles of medical ethics, cases we have identified challenge that assumption. Similarly, the results of those disclosures, including bedside interrogations by police and other state authorities, likely contradict most medical patients' expectations of privacy and humane treatment.[12]

Clinicians and trainees need to understand the ethical violations associated with breaches of patient confidentiality and trust, as well as their consequences. Providers' reports have been implicated in cases where a pregnant woman's search for healthcare has been met with coerced, forced, and unnecessary treatment; family separation; and incarceration, including detention in jails and healthcare facilities.[13] Furthermore, the fear of such consequences deters pregnant women from seeking needed healthcare (including prenatal and postpartum care, treatment for mental health and substance use disorders, and possibly even for conditions like diabetes and hypertension) and from confiding in and trusting their healthcare providers when they do so.

In this chapter, we describe the breaches themselves, the contexts in which they occur, and the harms they cause. We also recommend specific ways that providers can fulfill their commitment to nonmaleficence and respect for the patient's right to privacy and respond ethically to their pregnant patients,

including in conditions of moral distress (i.e., where institutional, procedural, or social constraints impede efforts to do the right thing). We hope to
complicate the thinking of healthcare providers who might be tempted to report a pregnant patient to authorities out of concern for unborn life or some
other reason without realizing the harm they are causing to the patient and
to the public's health and that such an action fuels a larger political project
to strip women and people with the capacity for pregnancy of fundamental
rights and personhood.[14]

The Breaches

Why do some healthcare professionals violate the privacy rights of pregnant patients? We surmise that a range of factors are at work. Some clinicians
overestimate the control a pregnant person has over a pregnancy outcome,
conflate a risk of harm with harm, or have an inflated sense of the degree of
risk of harm that an individual's actions pose to the pregnancy she carries.[15]
Healthcare providers and trainees are among those who may assign an
inordinate amount of blame to the consumption of *any* amount of a controlled substance despite the lack of scientific evidence that substances like
cannabis, cocaine, or opioids cause inevitable and irreversible harms to the
fetus.[16] Many of the effects (mis)attributed to substances frequently occur in
pregnancies in women who have preexisting (and previously undiagnosed)
conditions like heart disease or hypertension or who are burdened with the
weathering effects of chronic stress.[17] Providers also may underestimate or
neglect to communicate the seriousness of the risks associated with other
drugs, including prescription medications.[18]

Some providers may have reservations about breaching patient confidentiality but nonetheless comply with law enforcement requests or demands because, as we explain later, they incorrectly assume they must. Still others may
have a "knee jerk reaction" and defer to law enforcement officials without
pausing to consider whether such disclosure is required or the consequences
of such a disclosure for the patient. Healthcare providers, like other members
of the public, may subscribe to damaging stereotypes about people who
use drugs and be misinformed about the consequences of reporting a patient to the police and child welfare workers.[19] They may assume that mobi-
lizing authorities will yield supportive services rather than family separation,
stigma, and punishment.[20]

Healthcare providers' disclosures take a variety of forms and run a gamut in terms of the extent of provider initiative and involvement. Some health-care providers' disclosures occur in response to civil child welfare laws that address pregnancy and drug use as evidence of potential or actual (civil) child abuse or neglect. Many of these breaches reflect providers' misinfor-mation about or misunderstanding of what such laws actually require. Many cases—but by no means all—involve some claim of alleged harm or risk of harm due to substance use. Around 25 states and the District of Columbia have laws that require healthcare workers (acting as mandated reporters) to report to child welfare authorities if they suspect a person has used *any* amount of any controlled substance during pregnancy.[21] In many states, in-cluding New York and New Jersey, reporting takes place even though state law does not actually mandate such reporting.

In addition to these specific state laws, there is federal legislation, the Child Abuse Prevention and Treatment Act (CAPTA), that addresses the issue of pregnancy and drug use in a civil child welfare context. In order for states to receive certain federal dollars, CAPTA's provisions require "pol-icies and procedures (including appropriate referrals to child protection service systems and for other appropriate services) to address the needs of infants born with and identified as being affected by substance abuse or with-drawal symptoms resulting from prenatal drug exposure, or a Fetal Alcohol Spectrum Disorder."

CAPTA provides a directive to states, not to hospitals or healthcare providers. Moreover, it does not require states to have laws mandating re-porting based only on a positive toxicology (of either mother or infant) or a known history of substance use.[22] It addresses only newborns identi-fied as "affected" by substance abuse or those who experience withdrawal symptoms. This reporting does not need to take the form of an allegation of child abuse. The federal law simply requires a notification for purposes of connecting certain children to appropriate services. Nevertheless, this law is often referenced as justification for breaches of confidentiality that are not actually required.

Some disclosures stem from providers acting as vigilantes and contacting the police or child protective services on their own initiative, beyond any responsibilities as mandated reporters. For example, an Iowa mother went to the hospital after she fell down a flight of stairs while pregnant.[23] She and her pregnancy were fine. Medical staff, however, believing she might have been trying to end her pregnancy, contacted the police. As a result, when the woman left the hospital to return home to her two daughters, she was arrested on charges of attempted feticide. Women who have sought help at hospitals after a miscarriage, stillbirth, or an attempt to have an abortion have also found themselves subject to bedside interrogations and arrests because a hospital staff person (typically without any legal obligation to do so) reported them to authorities.[24]

Sometimes the disclosure originates with an actual, formal collaboration between hospital staff and law enforcement. In 1988, staff members at a public hospital operated by the Medical University of South Carolina established a collaborative policy with law enforcement. Hospital workers, in the guise of medical testing, searched pregnant women for evidence of drug use without a warrant or consent to a search for law enforcement purposes. They then turned that information over to the police along with other highly personal medical information and helped police carry out the arrests. In 2001, the US Supreme Court ruled in *Ferguson v. City of Charleston* that this collaboration violated patients' Fourth Amendment right to be free from unreasonable search and seizure.[25]

As this is written in 2020, hundreds of expectant and new mothers seeking care in hospitals in certain Alabama counties have been and continue to be drug tested without informed or specific consent, despite the fact that healthcare providers no doubt understand that the results will be reported to state authorities and lead to arrest under a radical judicial reinterpretation of the state's Chemical Endangerment of a Child law.[26] The 2006 law was passed to punish adults who brought children to dangerous places such as methamphetamine labs. The Alabama Supreme Court, however, ruled that the word "child" includes the unborn from the moment of fertilization and that a pregnant person's womb can be thought of as a dangerous environment, thus empowering law enforcement officials to use the law to arrest anyone who becomes pregnant and uses any amount of a controlled substance.[27] Arrests have included a woman who used half a tab of Valium, women who were receiving physician-prescribed methadone treatment, and a woman who used marijuana because she considered it to be a safer alternative to epilepsy medications with known risks to fetuses. More than 500 women have been arrested, many as a result of reports from hospital personnel who had no legal obligation to drug test and report pregnant women and new mothers.

On occasion, there may be a medically indicated reason why a provider wants to know about recent substance use. For example, if a patient is unconscious or otherwise unable to communicate, it might be helpful to determine if their status is caused or aggravated by substances, especially in an environment of widespread fentanyl contamination. There may be other limited medical reasons to test—with specific and informed consent that includes the possible social and legal consequences of a positive result—and use this information to support clinical care. Problems arise, however, when test results (including ones intended to be used only for diagnostic reasons) are accessed by other healthcare providers and social workers who view them as evidence of improper or criminal behavior.

Occasions where no medical reason exists, where testing takes place without specific and meaningful informed consent, and where test results and other private patient information are reported to law enforcement and others with the power to punish are among those that should evoke clinicians' and trainees' strong concern.[28] Registered neonatal NICU nurse and former National Perinatal Association board member Joelle Puccio also reminds providers that, "If you have a trusting relationship with your patients, you don't need to drug test because you can just ask the person what they took."[29]

People who have voluntarily sought help from healthcare providers have been reported to government authorities and then locked up or detained in mental hospitals and county jails or forced to submit to certain forms of treatment.[30] In 1998, Wisconsin enacted Wisconsin Act 292. This law, also known as the "Unborn Child Protection Act" or the "cocaine mom" law, purported to address problems associated with women who become pregnant and demonstrate a "habitual lack of self-control in the use of" alcohol or a controlled substance in a manner that creates "a substantial risk that the physical health of the unborn child, and of the child when born, will be seriously affected or endangered."[31] The Wisconsin law does not require healthcare providers to test or report women for evidence of pregnancy and alcohol or drug use. This law, however, does permit state authorities to lock a woman up and subject her to inappropriate and unconsented to medical treatment if she is pregnant and suspected of using or has disclosed *past* use of any amount of alcohol or a controlled substance.

Medical staff and state actors have transformed a person's efforts to obtain medical care into the basis for forced, unnecessary treatment and then incarceration. For example, Tamara Loertscher, a 29-year-old white woman in Wisconsin, had no health insurance and could not afford treatment for the severe thyroid problem she had had ever since she was a teenager. In 2014, she realized she might be pregnant. She went to a hospital seeking help and alternatives to the controlled substances she used for a short time to self-medicate for the depression and lethargy associated with severe hypo-thyroidism.[32] Instead, hospital staff focused on her past drug use and gave her confidential medical information to state authorities under Wisconsin Act 292. Court hearings were held to determine whether Ms. Loertscher could be deprived of her freedom. A lawyer was assigned to represent her 14-week fetus, but not Ms. Loertscher herself. A judge ordered Ms. Loertscher to jail, where she remained for 17 days, was denied prenatal care, kept off of her hypothyroid medication for two days, and spent three days in solitary confinement—all under the auspices of protecting an "unborn child."

"I was trying to do the right thing to take care of my pregnancy," Ms. Loertscher has said. "I was really sick when I went to get help, but I feel like asking for help just made everything worse."

The Harms

Provider disclosures to the police undermine the medical ethical commitment to patient privacy. They also violate the ethical principle of nonmaleficence that is captured in the popularized expression "do no harm." While providers may not intend to do harm, the individual and cumulative impact of their actions is often devastating to the pregnant patient. These disclosures often result in punitive responses that have serious social, legal, and public health consequences. Highly sensitive medical information has ended up not only in the hands of prosecutors and courts but also in full public view. Media coverage may range from a single story in the local press to extensive and ongoing coverage locally and nationally. Mugshots wind up on local newspaper circulars, on television, and all over the Internet. News stories may report drug use, employment history, sexually transmitted infections, and other potentially embarrassing or stigmatizing information. Women report humiliation, stress, and the loss of their jobs, custody of their children, and their reputations. A pregnant woman prosecuted under Alabama's chemical endangerment described at the time, "I feel like everywhere I go, people just kind of look at me and shame me like I'm a monster."[33] Her case was later dismissed.

When a pregnant patient being treated for an opioid use disorder with methadone or buprenorphine gives birth, the healthcare providers caring for the patient at the time of delivery may inform or be directed by state health authorities to inform the child welfare system, irrespective of how the patient is doing clinically. The same interpretation does not apply, however, to other prescribed medications, such as antidepressants and antiepileptics, that may also result in neonatal withdrawal syndromes. As the authors of a *Health Affairs* commentary observe, this approach "singles out newborns of women with opioid use disorder and perpetuates stigma toward the use of effective, life-saving medications such as methadone or buprenorphine."[34]

Violations of pregnant patients' rights to privacy in medical and personal information also lead to further violations of rights to physical liberty, informed consent and medical decision-making, bodily integrity, substantive and procedural due process, and protection from cruel and unusual punishment.[35] As mentioned earlier, efforts to establish separate legal "personhood" for fertilized eggs, embryos, and fetuses are being used as the basis for the arrests and detentions of and forced interventions on pregnant women, including those who seek to go to term. These threaten all pregnant women and people with the capacity for pregnancy not only with the loss of their reproductive rights and physical liberty but also with the loss of their status as full constitutional persons.[36] As explained in *American Journal of Public Health* commentary, pregnant women have been deprived of their liberty

> not only through the criminal justice system, but also through civil commitment proceedings and actions taken pursuant to civil child welfare laws. Pregnant women have been held in locked psychiatric wards and in treatment programs under 24-hour guard. They have been forced to undergo intimate medical examinations and blood transfusions over their religious objections. Women have been forced to submit to cesarean surgery, and some have been physically restrained with leather wrist and ankle cuffs so that they could be subjected to medical procedures they opposed.[37]

Providers' violations of their patients' privacy and collusion with law enforcement disclosures also undermine the health of new and expecting mothers and their families. Pregnant women and new mothers face sanctions and other consequences inflicted by criminal legal and child welfare systems that are harsh, dysfunctional, and target low-income people and people of color.[38] Parents have been separated from their newborns, lost custody of other children, been arrested, and faced stiff prison sentences as well as fines and court fees. Involuntary family separation causes significant trauma to children and their parents whether it occurs as a consequence of child welfare involvement or a parent's detention or incarceration.[39]

The price of these breaches is borne by the same people who are most susceptible to overpolicing and being ensnared in a criminal legal system that is extremely punitive. Black women are particularly likely to be reported to law enforcement and other state authorities by a healthcare provider. As physicians and nurses become more entangled in law enforcement, "the more they resemble agents of the police (and police informants and probation officers) rather than health care professionals."[40] Such entanglement erodes public trust in the "helping professions" of medicine and social work and diminishes public perceptions of hospitals as a site of humane and compassionate, patient-centered care. This trust is already fragile among many black, Indigenous, Latinx/Latine, immigrant, and low-income communities given experiences of forced sterilization, gynecological and other medical experimentation, and other occasions of medical racism.[41]

Fear of provider disclosure creates a climate where providers and patients regard one another with mutual distrust.[42] This suspicion deters many people from communicating openly and honestly with healthcare professionals and social workers who might be able to help them. It also deters people from seeking healthcare they need, including prenatal care and treatment for trauma (even when it is available). A Texas woman, convicted of a felony after giving birth to healthy twins, observed, "If I would have known that I'd get in trouble for telling my doctor the truth [that I was using cannabis to calm nausea], I would have either lied or not gone to the doctor."[43]

Medical staff mobilization of law enforcement can also have fatal consequences. In 2013, Jamie Lynn Russell, 33, went to an Oklahoma hospital in agonizing pain. Hospital staff perceived her as "noncompliant" (she was in too much pain to lie down) so they asked a police officer to assist. When police allegedly found that Ms. Russell had prescription pain pills that didn't belong to her, they took her to jail on charges of drug possession. Within two hours of being behind bars, Ms. Russell died of a ruptured ectopic pregnancy.[44]

What Can Be Done

Recognizing their ethical duties as well as the harms associated with providers participating in criminalizing and punitive processes, public health and medical organizations have long been united in their opposition to the use of punishment as a mechanism for addressing health concerns during pregnancy, including a person's use of criminalized substances. An AMA policy statement explicitly asserts that "Transplacental drug transfer should not be subject to criminal sanctions or civil liability."[45] The American College of Obstetrics and Gynecology (ACOG) Committee on Underserved Women also unequivocally states that "Seeking obstetric-gynecologic care should not expose a woman to criminal or civil penalties," including incarceration or loss of custody of her children.[46]

The ethical commitment to nonmaleficence challenges healthcare providers to address the sources of harm that are caused by systemic, institutional, and provider responses to pregnant patients. Professional associations should organize robust, empirically sound education programs that respect the complexity surrounding substance use, mental health, parenting, and pregnancy.[47] Providers should insist that policies and practice are grounded in science and evidence and principles of patient-centered health care, not sensationalism or stereotypes.[48]

Providers should ensure that policies and practices demonstrate an understanding of and respect for patients' privacy rights. When designing or weighing in on legislation or internal hospital policies to address issues relating to pregnancy, drug use, and treatment, healthcare providers should reject unethical legal mandates and internal hospital policies, including those that would expect evidence of past or present substance use to be reported as child abuse.

In the intimacy of the medical encounter, a patient may indicate their need or wish for more resources, social support, or medical care in many ways, including confiding in past drug use or using drugs during pregnancy. Reporting these patients through criminal and civil child abuse channels is more likely to cause additional harm. There are ways, however, that concerned clinicians can actually help their patients.

1. States can and should use CAPTA funds to develop a myriad of ways to offer services and support to families after a baby has been identified as drug affected and withdrawing, outside of the context of a punitive child neglect investigation and proceeding.[49] As long as CAPTA remains in effect, healthcare providers should do everything to ensure that newborns who need support for any reason can get it (e.g., from their communities or the government) rather than be reported to authorities.

2. Healthcare providers should know the foreseeable and harmful consequences of their actions should they report their pregnant patients to state authorities. Medical organizations should arrange and require that mandated reporters spend time observing family court proceedings so that they become better acquainted with the actual functioning of the child welfare system and the lack of resources and services available to struggling families and the pregnant patients and new mothers they might be tempted to report. Information about the possible consequences of a positive drug test result, for instance, should be integrated into specific and meaningful informed consent procedures. There must be no penalty for refusing to give consent to a test or procedure and no hospital policies penalizing hospital staff for respecting patient refusals.

3. Questionable or unethical laws, policies, and practices must be identified as such and challenged. The AMA Code of Ethics preamble recognizes that "[i]n some cases, the law mandates conduct that is ethically unacceptable." The Code states that "When physicians believe a law violates ethical values or is unjust, they should work to change the law." The ACOG Committee on Underserved Women similarly urges physicians to work with policymakers and legislators to retract punitive mandatory reporting policies and laws. Healthcare professionals should address their complicity in criminalizing processes and speak out as individuals and through their professional organizations and licensing boards and encourage others to do so as well (e.g., by participating in sign-on letters and amicus briefs, publishing commentaries, etc.).[50] Medical professionals who publish research should consider its social and political implications, including how it will be heard and understood in a culture marked by persistent racism, misogyny, and stigma against people who use criminalized substances or have a mental health problem.[51]

The ANA Provision 3.5 states that

nurses must be alert to and must take appropriate action in all instances of . . . practice or actions that place the rights or best interests of the patient in jeopardy or otherwise threaten the welfare of the patient, including reporting to authorities within the institution. If an ethically problematic practice continues to jeopardize patient well-being and safety, nurses must report the problem to appropriate external authorities such as practice committees of professional organizations, licensing boards, and regulatory or quality assurance agencies.

It is worth noting that the only place the ANA Code mentions law enforcement is in the context of reporting "especially egregious" situations and health care practices.

4. Pregnant patients deserve no fewer rights or guarantees of accuracy of testing than hospital workers and job applicants. If healthcare institutions do drug test pregnant patients, they cannot deprive them of procedures to ensure accuracy and fairness.[52] If a healthcare institution decides to conduct routine alcohol and drug testing, it should adopt the standards of federal workplace drug testing guidelines that establish certain cutoff levels to establish a true positive result and require confirmatory testing.

5. The AMA Code of Ethics states that "In exceptional circumstances of unjust laws, ethical responsibilities should supersede legal duties."[53] The arrests and prosecutions of people with the capacity for pregnancy arguably poses such an exceptional circumstance. Healthcare providers employed in states that expect them to report their pregnant patients to the police or child welfare authorities should consider civil disobedience. If doctors and nurses work in a state or in a hospital that treats a positive drug test result as evidence of child abuse, they should refuse to drug test their patients unless there is a clear clinically indicated reason to do so.

The AMA Code of Ethics states that, while caring for a patient, a physician shall "regard responsibility to the patient as paramount." People who seek medical attention for any aspect of pregnancy—including prenatal and postpartum care, labor and delivery, miscarriage, stillbirth, or abortion—should not fear arrest. The harmful practice of reporting patients to the police in the name of "protecting the unborn" needs to stop. At the end of the day, the soundest recommendation is also the most basic: If ordered or pressured by law enforcement officials, a colleague, or anyone else to violate fundamental principles of medical ethics and the rights and dignity of their pregnant patients, healthcare providers should follow the example set by nurse Alex Wubbels and the hospital where she worked: Speak up, and defend the patient.[54]

References

1. The authors would like to thank Hytham Imseis, MD (Novant Health Maternal-Fetal Medicine, Charlotte, NC), the editors, and an anonymous reviewer for their helpful comments on this chapter. An earlier version of this chapter was previously published in Flavin J, Paltrow LM. "Do no harm" like you mean it: Hospital workers' role in the policing of pregnant women. *Scholar & Feminist.* 2019;15(3), http://sfonline.barnard. edu/unraveling-criminalizing-webs-building-police-free-futures/do-no-harm-like-you-mean-it-hospital-workers-role-in-the-policing-of-pregnant-women/

2. Hawkins D. "This is crazy," sobs Utah hospital nurse as cop roughs her up, arrests her for doing her job. *Washington Post.* 2017 Sep 2. A few months later, Wubbels reached a $500,000 settlement with Salt Lake City; see Manson P. Utah nurse reaches $500,000 settlement in dispute over her arrest for blocking cop from drawing blood from patient. 2017 Oct 31, https://www.sltrib.com/news/2017/10/31/utah-nurse-arrested-for-blocking-cop-from-drawing-blood-from-patient-receives-500000-settlement/

3. A few years later, in 2020, another registered nurse, Dawn Wooten, made the news when she filed a complaint alleging that Spanish-speaking women detained at a private Georgia detention center were subjected to a disturbingly high rate of hysterectomies; many did not fully understand why they had undergone the procedure, calling attention to serious violations of principles of informed consent for medical procedures in the facility; see Paul K. ICE detainees faced medical neglect and hysterectomies, whistleblower alleges. *The Guardian.* 2020 Sep 14.

4. American Medical Association. Chapter 3: Opinions on privacy, confidentiality & medical records. Principles of Medical Ethics, https://www.ama-assn.org/delivering-care/privacy-health-care

5. American Nurses Association (ANA). *Code of Ethics for Nurses with Interpretive Statements.* 2015; Silver Spring, MD: ANA; 2015:10; Winland-Brown J, Lachman VD, Swanson EO. The new "Code of Ethics for Nurses with Interpretive Statements": Practical clinical application, Part I. *MEDSURG Nurs.* 2015;24(4):268–71.

6. American Medical Association. Chapter 3: Opinions on privacy, confidentiality & medical records.

7. Winland-Brown, Lachman, Swanson. Code of ethics for nurses with interpretive statements.

8. See Kohlman RJ. Unauthorized disclosure of confidential patient information, *Am Jur Trials.* 2020;32:105 (originally published in 1985; last updated Oct 2020); Zelin JE, Physician's tort liability for unauthorized disclosure of confidential information about patient. *A Law Rev.* 1986;48(4):668 (originally published in 1986; updated weekly); see also *Ferguson v. City of Charleston,* 532 U.S. 67 (2001); *Ferguson v. City of Charleston,* 308 F.3d 380 (4th Cir. 2002).

9. A note on our choice of language: historically, the state has targeted people identified as women for discrimination and state control based on pregnancy and their capacity for pregnancy. The overwhelming majority of people whom NAPW has represented and advocated for (and all of those identified in our earlier study) have been identified in public records as women. We recognize, of course, that not all people with

the capacity for pregnancy identify as women and that the gender binary itself contributes to systems of discrimination and control. Indeed, the larger project of reproductive justice contributes to an all-encompassing fight for civil and human rights (i.e., a true personhood movement). With this in mind, we variously use the terms "women," "pregnant people," and "people with the capacity for pregnancy" in recognition of the fact that all people are entitled to dignity, equality, and fairness regardless of gender identity, capacity for pregnancy, pregnancy, or stage of pregnancy including labor and delivery. Paltrow LM, Flavin J. Arrests of and forced interventions on pregnant women in the United States, 1973–2005: Implications for women's legal status and public health *J Health Politics Policy Law*. 2013;38(2):299–343, doi.org/10.1215/03616878-1966324.

10. Paltrow LM. Pregnant drug users, fetal persons, and the threat to *Roe v. Wade*. *Albany Law Rev*. 1999;62:999–1055.

11. Paltrow, Flavin. Arrests of and forced interventions on pregnant women in the United States, 1973–2005.

12. Ibid. See also Perritt J. #WhiteCoatsForBlackLives—Addressing physicians' complicity in criminalizing communities. *N Engl J Med*. 2020;383(19):1804–6.

13. For instance, in Florida, a pregnant woman was held prisoner at the hospital and forced to have caesarean surgery. The baby was stillborn. See Belkin L. Is refusing bedrest a crime? *New York Times* 2010 Jan 12, https://parenting.blogs.nytimes.com/2010/01/12/is-refusing-bed-rest-a-crime?mtrref=undefined

14. Movement for Family Power. 2020. "Whatever they do, I'm her protector." How the foster system has become ground zero for the drug war. 2020 Jun, https://www.movementforfamilypower.org/ground-zero Perritt. #WhiteCoatsForBlackLives.

15. Minkoff H, Marshall MF. Fetal risks, relative risks, and relatives' risks. *Am J Bioethics*. 2016; 6(2):3–11, doi:10.1080/15265161.2015.1120791.

16. Torres CA, Medina-Kirchner C, O'Malley KY, Hart CL. Totality of the evidence suggests prenatal cannabis exposure does not lead to cognitive impairments: A systematic and critical review. *Front Psychol*. 2020;11:816, doi: 10.3389/fpsyg.2020.00816; Frank DA, Augustyn M, Knight WG, Pell T, Zuckerman B. Growth, development, and behavior in early childhood following prenatal cocaine exposure: A systematic review. *JAMA* 2001;285:1613–25; Wright TE, Schuetter R, Tellei J, Sauvage L. Methamphetamines and pregnancy outcomes. *J Addiction Med*. 2015;9(2):111–17, doi:10.1097/ADM.0000000000000101; Smith LM, Diaz S, LaGasse LL, et al. Developmental and behavioral consequences of prenatal methamphetamine exposure: A review of the Infant Development, Environment, and Lifestyle (IDEAL) study. *Neurotoxicol Teratol*. 2015;51:35–44, doi:10.1016/j.ntt.2015.07.006; Van Boekel LC, Brouwers EPM, Weeghel J, Garretsen HFL. Stigma among health professionals towards patients with substance use disorders and its consequences for healthcare delivery: Systematic review. *Drug Alcohol Dependence*. 2013;131(1–2):23–35, https://doi.org/10.1016/j.drugalcdep.2013.02.018; Sunderlin K, Huss L. The mythology of "addicted babies": Challenging media distortions, laws, and policies that fracture communities. *DifferenTakes* 2014; issue paper 86, http://hdl.handle.net/10009/939; Flavin J,

Paltrow LM. Punishing pregnant drug-using women: Defying law, medicine, and common sense. *J Addictive Dis.* 2010;29:231–44.

17. Preexisting chronic medical conditions (such as hypertension, diabetes, and heart disease) play a substantial role in the health of pregnant women and pregnancy outcomes, as do preexisting social conditions. See The Stillbirth Collaborative Research Network Writing Group. Causes of death among stillbirths. *JAMA.* 2011;306(22):2459–68; Gordon C, Smith, S, Pell JP. Cesarean section and risk of unexplained stillbirth in subsequent pregnancy. *Lancet.* 2003;362:1779–84; Cnattingius S, Stephansson O. The epidemiology of stillbirth. *Semin Perinatol.* 2002;26:25–30; Eller AG, Byrne JLB. Stillbirth at term. *Obstet Gynecol.* 2006;108(2):442–7; Zotti, ME, Williams AM, Robertson M, Horney J, Hsia J. Post-disaster reproductive health outcomes. *Maternal Child Health J.* 2013;17(5):783–96, https://doi-org.avoserv2.library.fordham.edu/10.1007/s10995-012-1068-x; Scorza P, Monk C. Anticipating the stork: Stress and trauma during pregnancy and the importance of prenatal parenting, zero to three. 2019;39(5):5–13; Zero to Three IS the journal title. See: https://www.bluetoad.com/publication/?i=589447&p=1&pp=1&view=issueViewer; Geronimus AT. The weathering hypothesis and the health of African-American women and infants: Evidence and speculations. *Ethnicity Dis.* 1992;2(3):207–21. Many of the intrauterine stressors that are thought to have adverse intergenerational effects "correlate with social gradients of class, race and gender." Miranda ML, Maxson P, Edwards S. Environmental contributions to disparities in pregnancy outcomes. *Epidemiol Rev.* 2009;31(1):67–83, p. 68; Richardson SS, Daniels CR, Gillman MW, Golden J, Kukla R, Kuzawa C, Rich-Edwards J. Don't blame the mothers. *Nature.* 2014;512:131–2; Flavin, Paltrow. Punishing pregnant drug-using women.

18. Wakeman SE, Jordan A, Beletsky L. When reimagining systems of safety, take a closer look at the child welfare system. *Health Affairs.* 2020 Oct 7, https://www.healthaffairs.org/do/10.1377/hblog20201002.72121/full/; Movement for Family Power. "Whatever they do, I'm her protector."

19. Perritt. #WhiteCoatsForBlackLives;. Van Boekel et al. Stigma among health professionals towards patients with substance use disorders.

20. Movement for Family Power. "Whatever they do, I'm her protector"; Perritt. #WhiteCoatsForBlackLives.

21. Guttmacher Institute. State policies on substance use during pregnancy. Guttmacher Institute. 2020, https://www.guttmacher.org/state-policy/explore/substance-use-during-pregnancy

22. Price A, Bergin C, Little C, et al. Implementing child abuse prevention and treatment act (CAPTA) requirements to serve substance-exposed newborns: Lessons from a collective case study of four program models. *J Public Child Welfare* [serial online]. 2012 Apr 1;6(2):149–71; National Advocates for Pregnant Women. Understanding CAPTA and state obligations. Fact sheet. 2020 Oct 29, https://www.nationaladvocatesforpregnantwomen.org/understanding-capta-and-state-obligations/

23. Newman A. Iowa "feticide" law could be used to target mothers. *Huffington Post.* 2010 Apr 18, https://www.huffingtonpost.com/amie-newman/iowa-feticide-law-could-b_b_463153.html

24. The Editorial Board. How my stillbirth became a crime. *New York Times*. Video. 2018 Dec 28, https://www.nytimes.com/interactive/2018/12/28/opinion/stillborn-murder-charge.html

25. 2001.532 U.S. 67 *Ferguson v. City of Charleston*, 532 U.S. 67 (2001); *Ferguson v. City of Charleston*, 308 F.3d 380 (4th Cir. 2002).

26. Martin N. How some Alabama hospitals quietly drug test new mothers— without their consent. 2015 Sep 30, https://www.propublica.org/article/how-some-alabama-hospitals-drug-test-new-mothers-without-their-consent; see also Martin N. Alabama mom's charges dropped, but only after an arduous battle. ProPublica. 2016 Jun 6, https://www.propublica.org/article/alabama-moms-charges-are-dropped-but-only-after-an-arduous-battle

27. National Advocates for Pregnant Women. Press statement. National Advocates for Pregnant Women's Lynn Paltrow on Alabama Supreme Court's decision in "personhood" measure in disguise case. 2013 Jan 12, https://www.nationaladvocatesfor pregnantwomen.org/press-statement-national-advocates-for-pregnant-womens-lynn-paltrow-on-alabama-supreme-courts-decision-in-personhood-measure-in-disguise-case/

28. ACOG guidelines on drug testing stipulate that providers should provide patients with information about what could happen if the test is positive. In reality, not all hospitals make it clear that when patients sign consent forms they are consenting to a drug test or how results will be used. Language about the testing may be buried in general consent paperwork; people in active labor, in particular, might not read or consider the consent forms carefully. Hospital admissions consent forms that patients are expected to sign at admission may describe a wide range of hospital policies, including a statement that the hospital may perform unspecified laboratory tests "when appropriate." Such admissions forms typically fail to inform pregnant patients that they may be tested for drugs or of the consequences of a positive drug test result (i.e., that a positive drug test result may trigger arrest and prosecution or child welfare involvement). Martin, Yurkanin. How some Alabama hospitals quietly drug test new mothers.

29. Puccio also notes that, "In my 15 years, I have only once seen a tox screen that was used for clinical purposes. They are ordered and used for the primary purpose of providing evidence either for or against the patient." Puccio J. Personal communication and used here with permission; 2018 Sep 19.

30. Eckholm E. Case explores rights of fetus versus mother. *New York Times* 2014 Oct 24, http://www.nytimes.com/2013/10/24/us/case-explores-rights-of-fetus-versus-mother.html. See also "The Case of Alicia Beltran." Video, https://vimeo.com/202241357

31. 1997 Wisconsin Act 292, codified as Wis. Stat. § 48.133 et seq.

32. Vielmetti B. Pregnant woman challenging Wisconsin protective custody law. *Milwaukee Journal-Sentinel*. 2015 Jan 2, http://www.jsonline.com/news/wisconsin/pregnant-woman-challenging-wisconsin-protective-custody-law-b99411705z1-287395241.html

33. Martin N. Take a Valium, lose your kid, go to jail. *Digg*. 2015 Sep 23, http://digg.com/2015/alabama-drug-laws-pregnant-women

34. Wakeman, Jordan, Beletsky. When reimagining systems of safety.

35. Paltrow LM. *Roe v Wade* and the New Jane Crow: Reproductive rights in the age of mass incarceration. *AJPH*. 2013;103(1):17–21. doi:10.2105/AJPH.2012.301104.

36. Ibid.

37. Ibid. Citations removed; can be found in the original article.

38. See also Roberts D. *Killing the Black Body*. New York: Random House; 1998; Roberts D. *Shattered Bonds: The Color of Child Welfare*. New York: Basic Books; 2002; Perritt. #WhiteCoatsForBlackLives.

39. Turney K, Wildeman C. Maternal incarceration and the transformation of urban family life. *Social Forces* 2018; (3):1155–82;Roberts. *Shattered Bonds*; Lee T. *Catching a Case: Inequality and Fear in New York City's Child Welfare System*. New Brunswick, NJ: Rutgers; 2016; Cloud E, Oyama R, Teichner L. Family defense in the age of Black Lives Matter. *CUNY Law Rev.* 2017;(20):68–94.

40. Annas GJ. *American Bioethics: Crossing Human Rights and Health Law Boundaries*. New York: Oxford University Press; 2005: 117.

41. Cooper-Owens D. *Medical Bondage: Race, Gender, and the Origins of American Gynecology*. Athens, GA: University of Georgia Press; 2018; Washington H. *Medical Apartheid: The Dark History of Medical Experimentation on Black Americans from Colonial Times to the Present*. New York: Doubleday; 2006.

42. Roberts SC, Pies C. Complex calculations: How drug use during pregnancy becomes a barrier to prenatal care. *Matern Child Health J.* 2011;15(3):333–41. Stone R. Pregnant women and substance use: Fear, stigma, and barriers to care. *Health Justice*, 2015;3:2–15, http://doi.org/10.1186/s40352-015-0015-5; Roberts SCM, Nuru-Jeter A. Women's perspectives on screening for alcohol and drug use in prenatal care. *Women's Health Issues*. 2010;20(3):193–200, doi:10.1016/j.whi.2010.02.003.

43. Martin. Take a Valium.

44. Kemp A. Family of Pauls Valley woman who died in custody seeks answers. *The Oklahoman*. 2013 Feb 4, http://newsok.com/article/3751456

45. National Advocates for Pregnant Women. Medical and Public Health Group Statements Opposing Prosecution and Punishment of Pregnant Women (revised June 2018), https://www.nationaladvocatesforpregnantwomen.org/wp-content/uploads/2020/05/Medical-and-Public-Health-Group-Statements-revised-June-2018.pdf

46. The American College of Obstetricians and Gynecologists. Substance abuse reporting and pregnancy: The role of the obstetrician-gynecologist. Committee Opinion 473. *Obstet Gynecol.* 2011 Jan. 117:200–201 (reaffirmed 2014).

47. If one is qualified to offer such testimony, people should make themselves available to serve as an expert witness in cases involving the prosecution of pregnant women. For example, in the 2015 Indiana case of Purvi Patel, the defense introduced expert testimony to debunk that of the pathologist for the prosecution who relied on the "lung float test"—dating back from the seventeenth century and discredited more than 100 years ago—to argue that the fetus was born alive.

48. In this regard, interested readers are encouraged to consult the resources of the National Perinatal Association and the Academy of Perinatal Harm Reduction.

49. Price et al. Implementing child abuse prevention and treatment act (CAPTA) requirements.

50. Perritt. #WhiteCoatsForBlackLives.

51. Singer LT, Chambers C, Coles C, Kable J. Fifty years of research on prenatal substances: Lessons learned for the opioid epidemic. *J Res Pract.* 2020:1–12, doi:10.1007/s42844-020-00021-7. The moral panic over "crack babies" in the 1980s and 1990s was informed, in no small part, by the media attention surrounding a small and poorly designed study of 23 infants and the first author's overstatement of his findings. Chasnoff IJ, Burns WJ, Schnoll SH, Burns KA. Cocaine use in pregnancy. *N Engl J Med*; 1985;313:666–9. Chasnoff et al.'s study, and the hysteria that ensued, is documented in the *New York Times* Retro Reports video, "The Crack Epidemic That Wasn't." See also: From crack babies to Oxytots: Lessons not learned. Video, http://www.retroreport.org/video/from-crack-babies-to-oxytots-lessons-not-learned. Even today, researchers continue to frame their research questions and findings in careless or otherwise problematic ways. For example, Harvard researchers fielded a survey to more than 800 physicians in 21 states asking doctors about "their willingness to seek court intervention in an effort to compel maternal compliance when women fail to adhere to treatments that are recommended for fetal benefit." The article, including the abstract and summary, repeated the concept of "court intervention" or authorization to compel maternal compliance more than 20 times. No matter how discredited or ethically problematic an idea is, if it is repeated often enough, it can gain legitimacy and currency. Through dint of repetition, the article presents these problematic notions as apparently valid and normative ones. Brown SD, Donelan K, Martins Y, et al., Differing attitudes toward fetal care by pediatric and maternal-fetal medicine specialists. *Pediatrics.* 2012;130(6):e1534–e1540, doi:10.1542/peds.2012-1352. Positive examples also exist of findings presented in a way that contextualizes the social and political context of the research; see Frank et al. Growth, development, and behavior in early childhood following prenatal cocaine exposure.

52. In 1993, the US Department of Health and Human Services Substance Abuse Mental Health Services Administration (SAMHSA) convened an expert consensus panel to address the issue of drug testing and specifically the question of whether or not pregnant women and new mothers should routinely be tested for evidence of drug use. While their findings recognized that certain criteria were used by some healthcare institutions to test some women, the panel did not recommend adopting any of these criteria nor did it endorse the routine drug testing of pregnant patients. They did recommend that if hospitals were going to test, they should do so pursuant to federal workplace drug testing guidelines. Mandatory Guidelines for Federal Workplace Drug Testing Program: Final Rule. *Federal Register.* 2017; 82:7920.

53. American Medical Association. 2016. "Preamble." Code of Medical Ethics Opinions, https://www.ama-assn.org/sites/default/files/media-browser/preface-and-preamble-to-opinions.pdf

54. Chappell B. Calling nurse a "hero," Utah hospital bars police from patient-care areas. National Public Radio. 2017 Sep 5, https://www.npr.org/sections/thetwo-way/2017/09/05/548601099/calling-nurse-a-hero-utah-hospital-bars-police-from-patient-care-areas

14

Prenatal Counseling for
Maternal–Fetal Surgery

Potential Biases, Competing Interests, and Undue Practice Variation in the World of Fetal Care

Stephen D. Brown MD

The fragility of crystal is not a weakness but a fineness.
—John Krakauer (Into the Wild)

More Choices, Weightier Decisions

In 1965, longtime *Pediatrics* editor and neonatologist Jerold Lucey suggested that successful direct fetal treatment would, for some, render indistinct the line between obstetrics and pediatrics.[1] This was the year that Sir William Liley published his landmark paper describing intrauterine fetal therapy for Rh incompatibility.[2] For Liley and other fetal therapy pioneers, the enticing possibilities created a self-perceived separate relationship with the fetus as the direct object of therapeutic intervention and physician obligation. Such a perception was associated with an expressed distinction between the fetus and pregnant woman, one in which the fetus was recognized as a new class of patient.[3,4] Direct intrauterine prenatal surgery has since become a real option in certain settings, with fetal spina bifida as its first demonstrated success, facilitated by technological developments in prenatal diagnosis, pediatric medicine, surgery, and obstetrics.[5-7] And, true to Lucey's vision, obstetrics, neonatology, and pediatrics more broadly have subsequently merged operations under a common paradigm of *fetal care.*[7-9]

Other medical and social developments concurrent with the evolution of fetal care have yielded an increasingly complex context within which clinical obstetrical decisions must be made. In 1973, abortion was legalized in the United States, tethered to a biometric parameter—viability—that became achievable at progressively earlier gestational ages.[10,11] Prenatal diagnostic technologies moved toward increasingly confident identification of conditions like Down syndrome and spina bifida, which accelerated termination rates for affected pregnancies.[12] Concomitant improvements in pediatric care and societal accommodations for people born with developmental and functional impairments enhanced their survival and life quality such that palliative postnatal care for babies diagnosed with conditions such as spina bifida and Down syndrome, once routine, became increasingly unacceptable.[5]

The confluence of these technological and cultural developments has created a new social category of prospective parents empowered with more choices during pregnancy when potentially treatable prenatal conditions are diagnosed. The array of available options presents patients and their physicians with ever-weightier ethical and communication challenges. Diametrically opposed management alternatives, such as abortion and intrauterine surgery, are now available for historically "lethal" and "nonlethal" fetal conditions, and both alternatives may be actionable at gestational ages where neonatal survival may be possible. Some intrauterine procedures carry considerable maternal and fetal/neonatal risks.[5,6,13] Prospective parents and clinicians alike must routinely assess the risks and benefits of available clinical options within the context of moral and religious values, socioeconomic considerations, social expectations, and complex emotions. Diagnostic certitude may be hard to reconcile with uncertainty of outcome. An expansive range of plausible scenarios may exist for a future child's developmental status, functional abilities, and medical needs across multiple organ systems. Clinical recommendations and parental decisions are commonly made under substantial time pressure because diagnosis and counseling often take place just before the legal limit on pregnancy termination has been reached and because certain prenatal therapies are performed within limited time windows.

Such decisions must also be made within the context of intense societal divisions around the appropriateness of pregnancy termination and the ethical responsibilities of pregnant women toward fetuses. As we shall see herein, such divisions may be manifest among providers from different specialties. To shield their patients from such tensions and any endemically embedded biases, the community of clinicians who provide prenatal counseling to pregnant women and their partners when these conditions are diagnosed remains steadfastly committed to maintaining a culture of value-neutral counseling.[14] This commitment assumes a prima facia and empirically underexplored premise that unbiased counseling is really possible.

Crystal's Journey

Let us consider here a young woman named Crystal. She is 21 years old and 21 weeks pregnant. Unmarried and without a relationship with her former partner, she has nonetheless been excited by the pregnancy, the prospect of motherhood, and the surprisingly strong feelings she has already developed for the baby. Without concerns for her health, and because of her demanding work obligations (she holds two jobs), she presents late for her first detailed obstetrical ultrasound, which shows a male fetus with a lumbosacral myelomeningocele (spina bifida) and mildly enlarged cerebral ventricles, consistent with a brain malformation characteristic of the condition. Her primary obstetrician tells her that if the baby is born, he will need at least surgical repair of the spinal defect and likely a plastic shunt tunneled underneath the skin from the cranium into the abdomen to divert spinal fluid from his obstructed ventricles. Many additional surgeries and medical treatments may be necessary during his life, requiring an array of specialists including neonatologists, neurosurgeons, urologists, orthopedic surgeons, and developmental medicine pediatricians. Crystal is referred to multiple clinicians for prenatal counseling. She meets with a maternal–fetal medicine obstetrics specialist in a major general hospital and is then referred to a children's hospital's fetal care center, where, she is told, she may undergo further magnetic resonance imaging (MRI) and meet with a multidisciplinary team. Crystal's excitement turns to fear, confusion, and sadness because she doesn't know whether she can give this baby the care that it needs. She has always taken pride in her self-sufficiency, but now she is keenly more aware of her limited resources and social supports. Early on, she had dismissed thoughts about terminating the pregnancy, but now she is seriously considering the option.

As Crystal moves among specialists and institutions seeking information, guidance, and support, at issue is whether it is truly possible that she will receive value-neutral counseling washed clean of the myriad impressions, ethical and religious predilections, clinical interests and experiences, institutional priorities, and frank biases that may exist. As we explore the world

Crystal has entered, we shall see that it seems probable that such values and interests will creep unwittingly into the counseling she receives, such that their weight is felt and their influence seeps into her decision-making despite the veil of neutrality that has been constructed to protect her.

Facts and Values

At the least, Crystal's new world is not isolated from larger societal tensions existing around abortion. Within such morally controversial territory as reproductive decision-making, physicians hold variable self-perceived obligations regarding what information to convey or withhold and what referrals to make or services to offer.[15-20] Concern abounds that counseling about reproductive health matters—and, more importantly, outcomes— reflects an amalgam of facts and values that vary according to physician demographic characteristics such as age, gender, religion, and political ideology.

A complex interplay of facts and values has long suffused the world of counseling around complex prenatally diagnosed fetal conditions. Consider hypoplastic left heart syndrome (HLHS). Like many conditions once considered lethal, this severe heart condition is now survivable, often requiring multiple surgeries and prolonged intensive care, with diverse practice models and variable outcomes.[21,22] Providers remain divided regarding the appropriateness of various treatment alternatives, such as abortion, postnatal palliative care, staged surgical repair/palliation, and cardiac transplantation.[22-26] Many specialists' personal preferences regarding treatment have remained static despite longitudinal outcome improvements.[25] Many reportedly do not discuss all potential management options prenatally with patients, and they commonly recommend potential surgical options when they themselves would choose nontreatment or abortion.[24,25,27] Some providers may selectively suggest treatment alternatives available at their institutions or that they themselves perform without discussing outcomes elsewhere.[27] Certainly, some patients may self-refer to specific institutions wanting exclusively to hear about postnatal surgical alternatives and not abortion. Alternatively, some physicians may perceive this to be so, without knowing patients' actual preferences. Regardless, a troubling pattern of practice variation has emerged in which recommendations provided and decisions ultimately made may flow more from provider biases and disparate institutional interests than medical facts. Such practice variation has become common in obstetrics, pediatrics, and medicine generally and has raised broad concerns about whether patient preferences are systematically overpowered.[28]

The same problems exist in prenatal counseling for conditions that can be treated with intrauterine surgery, for which spina bifida is the paradigmatic example. Postnatal palliative care, once common, would now rarely be considered for a baby with spina bifida. Over the duration that abortion has been legal and prenatal diagnosis has been reliable, prenatal decision-making has been essentially binary. When diagnosed, either the pregnancies were terminated, or the spinal defects were repaired postnatally. As ethically challenging as these decisions were, the calculus became more complex in 2011, when a randomized trial was published of prenatal surgical repair.[29-31] Compared to babies who underwent postnatal repair, half as many who underwent prenatal repair required shunts by 12 months of age (40% vs. 82%), and twice as many walked independently at 30 months (42% vs. 21%). The trial was considered a success; in fact, it was stopped early according to prespecified metrics. A third option for prenatally diagnosed spina bifida thus became available. Compared to postnatal repair, however, prenatal repair is associated with important maternal morbidities. The intrauterine procedure currently entails open maternal laparotomy and a uterine fundal incision, with subsequent cesarean delivery via separate incision and a requirement for cesarean section in subsequent pregnancies. Rates of chorioamniotic separation, maternal pulmonary edema, oligohydramnios, placental abruption, maternal transfusion, and partial or complete uterine dehiscence are all significantly increased for women undergoing prenatal surgery. Neonatal morbidity and mortality are also higher.

As with postnatal surgery for HLHS, opinions among informed providers about prenatal surgery for fetal spina bifida have long been mixed.[4,8,13,32,33] A decade prior to the trial, one noted British neurosurgeon posited that, for intrauterine surgery to be acceptable, postnatal improvement would have to be substantially greater than was actually demonstrated in the trial.[33] Physician views post trial remain variable. Some have modified their positions about the various options for prenatally diagnosed spina bifida, although a 2014 Cochrane review of trials comparing prenatal and postnatal surgery found insufficient evidence to justify firm conclusions because only one such trial had been published and only a small number of pregnancies overall have been evaluated.[34,35] Some now hold the prenatal surgery as a new standard of care while others express reticence given ongoing maternal morbidity.[36-38] Physician views about the surgery will likely continue to vary even as the surgery becomes less maternally invasive and postnatal outcomes change.[8,39,40]

Professional Cultures and Lived Values

Beyond narrow surgical considerations, counseling clinicians have long held disparate attitudes about management alternatives for various prenatally diagnosed conditions.[41,42] As Crystal moves among different specialists for consultation, it seems evident that she will likely encounter specialists whose views and recommendations about prenatally diagnosed fetal conditions reflect an alchemy of diverse values around abortion, maternal obligations, physician obligations, and disability.[8,35,39,42-44] As with other realms of re-productive health, these physicians' ethical positions are often informed by important personal demographics, such as age, gender, religiosity, and po-litical orientation. But they are not removed from clinical experiences that may lead to divergent understandings of how conditions behave and the risks, benefits, burdens and rewards they create for patients and families.[42] Just as gender or age may be independently associated with clinicians' views about abortion, who should provide counseling and when, or what informa-tion and services should be discussed, so, too, may their experiences caring for children with disabilities or pregnant women across the spectrum of their respective social and medical experiences.

For dedicated and caring clinicians, the emotional power of these experiences may contribute to deeply held "lived values"—those which em-anate from "the actual practices and engagement of what really matters in a particular place and time among vexed patients, families, and clinicians."[45] Such lived values may influence physicians' self-perceived obligations to pregnant women, fetuses, and future children or these physicians' perceptions of how much physical risk, if any, pregnant women should as-sume for any given degree of benefit to the fetus or future child.[42] Physicians' experiences with pregnant women's particular psychosocial vulnerabilities may influence their attitudes regarding what burdens may reasonably be imposed upon these women's liberty interests. Similarly, physicians' engage-ment in the lives of individuals with congenital differences may sway how strongly the physicians advocate for these individuals' protections and their views about whether such advocacy extends to pregnancy-related decisions. Cognitive and ethical dissonance may arise when clinicians are asked to support decisions that run counter to the values that have been informed by their intensely lived clinical experiences. Such tensions may manifest differently among the obstetrics-based and pediatrics-based providers whom Crystal might meet.[8,35,39,42-44]

Furthermore, these specialists may function within distinct professional cultures where perspectives differ regarding the maternal–fetal relationship, the applicability of best interest standards to pregnancy-related decisions, and the ethical appropriateness of alternate management options.[28,46] Prior to the issuance in 2011 of joint guidelines of the American College of Obstetricians and Gynecologists (ACOG) and the American Academy of Pediatrics (AAP) regarding the ethics of maternal–fetal interventions, these separate professional organizations offered subtly divergent analyses of maternal autonomy, maternal and physician obligations, the psychosocial vulnerabilities faced by pregnant women, norms of directiveness, and the appropriateness of utilizing judicial authorization to override maternal refusal of physician recommendations.[46,47] Evidence suggests that such specialty differences are sometimes reflected at the individual provider level.[42] Ultimately, for patients like Crystal who are struggling with what to do when congenital conditions such as spina bifida, Down syndrome, or HLHS are prenatally identified, it is probable that the recommendations she hears from different physicians reflect an intricate fermentation process in which physicians' professional experiences and environments act independently adjacent to demographic variables (and clinical facts) to inform their ultimate views and recommendations.

Healthcare Delivery Systems for Fetal Care

Adding to the complexity for Crystal and her cohort, healthcare delivery systems for prenatally diagnosed conditions have evolved rapidly. A generation ago, prenatal counseling for such conditions was predominantly the domain of obstetrics-based practitioners, especially those specializing in maternal–fetal medicine and commonly practicing within either independent obstetrical units or those within larger general hospitals. The recent proliferation of fetal care centers often housed within pediatrics-based institutions and/ or under the leadership of pediatrics-based specialists has brought further heterogeneity into institutional organizational structures and practice models.[8,9] It is possible that variation in how these centers are structured leads to variation in prenatal counseling. Some fetal care centers exist within free-standing, independent children's hospitals with sophisticated facilities for imaging, prenatal surgery, delivery, and post-procedure recovery for both the pregnant women and their babies. Others are comprehensive health system partnerships in which obstetrics units within various hospitals (including Catholic hospitals that do not offer abortion counseling) refer directly into a dedicated pediatrics center with sophisticated prenatal services. One major children's hospital has acquired an extensive obstetrics practice network, such that a sizable, full-service reproductive care enterprise is now controlled by a pediatrics-based institution that also runs its own independent health plan.

These differences in practice models might result in counseling differences affecting how fetal surgery and abortion are presented or whether the options are presented at all. As has been seen with pediatric cardiac and neonatal care, differing operations and technological capabilities may themselves contribute strongly to practice variation.[21,28,48] Referral patterns and financial incentives may vary. Different centers may apply different inclusion criteria and have variable levels of experience and success with various procedures. State laws about abortion may affect institutions differently, and different institutions themselves may have variable abortion policies. Patients in states with restrictive abortion policies who receive care within obstetrics-based systems that have restrictive policies themselves and who refer internally within their systems for pediatrics-based fetal care may be counseled differently from patients in states where abortion law is more permissive and/or where obstetrics-based and pediatrics-based prenatal services are separately and independently controlled.

Where Does All This Leave Crystal?

Overall, the constellation of conditions Crystal will encounter during her journey closely resembles that within neonatal care, whereupon variable provider attitudes about such matters as what information should be dispensed and what decisions are ethically appropriate interact within heterogeneous delivery systems to create environments in which the management alternatives offered and recommendations made are informed as much by individual biases and differing institutional predilections as by facts.[48] The similarities between fetal care and neonatal care are striking, but not surprising. Both domains straddle the interface of obstetrics and pediatrics, where moral status is a technologically dependent target shifting unsteadily amid fluid social and political norms. As with HLHS, the experience in neonatology has raised prominent concerns that the specific locus of care—and even the specific provider at any given moment—may influence the information, options, recommendations, and directiveness of counseling; hold undue sway over the decisions patients (parents) make; and account for empirically untethered practice variation.[48]

For Crystal, and other pregnant patients seeking prenatal consultation after congenital conditions such as spina bifida, Down syndrome, or HLHS are identified, the portals to potential bias and practice variation in the counseling they receive are as gaping as for neonatology. As various individual biases and institutional interests compete to influence the ultimate counseling that occurs at the bedside, these windows will always be open. Human nature is too intransigent. Institutional idiosyncrasies are too powerful. The technology is too alluring. How can these patients know whether any given provider or center will differ from others in their endorsement of the options patients may choose? The information or services they make available? The pressure brought to bear? They can't. The windows are too opaque. As with neonatology, decision-making remains confined within "the dark recesses of [an] unlit landscape."[49]

Recommendations for Mitigating the Effects of Potential Bias and Competing Interests in Fetal Care

Greater transparency is necessary to help Crystal and patients like her understand better the complex world they have entered and how various biases and interests may compete with their own values and preferences in driving the decisions they must make. One mechanism to promote transparency would be to treat these circumstances as we would others where variables other than primary professional concerns about patients' interests exert undue influence over clinicians' behavior. Dennis Thompson, in his landmark 1993 paper on conflicts of interest, focused on financial conflicts not because they were more important than other conflicting interests, but rather because they were more objectively identifiable, measurable, and remediable.[50] Since then, a solid body of literature (much cited here) has provided a sound empirical foundation for understanding and quantifying how various other physician and institutional factors function similarly to classically understood financial conflicts in influencing the recommendations that physicians make and the services they may offer.

Given that various gateways to bias existing in fetal care are quantifiably evaluable and may function similarly to financial conflicts of interest in how they sway physician behavior, they merit similar standards of transparency and disclosure. Just as mechanisms now exist to inform patients and research subjects of financial relationships that may influence physicians' recommendations or the information they provide, similar vehicles could be established to educate patients about the various biases and competing interests that may color the prenatal counseling they receive. The AAP and ACOG recommend that independent patient advocates be offered to support pregnant women in their decision-making.[47] General literature-based or web-based resources could be provided that describe how biases may be embedded in counseling and referral processes. Information could be made readily available about how external laws or internal mandates may impact accessible services. Individual institutions could be compelled to offer transparent accounting of services they do and do not provide, how institutions differ elsewhere, their experience with various conditions and procedures, individual outcomes compared to outcomes elsewhere, and other variables that might influence their recommendations.[28] A database of services and outcomes across institutions could be constructed, with requirements similar to those for assisted reproductive technology, in which clinics are required by law to gather and report data on success rates in a standardized format so patients can compare. Additional information could be provided on whether obstetrics centers or insurance plans are tied operationally and financially to the pediatrics-based centers with which they are associated. Such resources could be augmented by published or electronic decision aids similar to those used in prenatal testing that guide patients toward identifying and articulating their unique preferences.[51] They would serve essentially as devices to enhance informed consent, empowering pregnant patients and their partners to ask more sophisticated questions and seek courses of action that most closely align with their needs and preferences.

Of course, individual counseling practitioners must be prepared to discuss these matters openly and honestly. Such preparation would first require reconsideration of norms regarding value-neutral counseling. Acknowledgment might be given to the reasonable likelihood that our veils of neutrality are simply too porous.[52] Although neutrality may protect patients from the influence of clinicians' values, it may also inhibit transparency and permit concerted biases to be transmitted more subtlety and unwittingly—through nuances of language; framing of risk, benefit, and outcomes; expressed support for various decisions; and/or services discussed and offered. A sustained critique within the genetic counseling literature has long asserted that nondirective prenatal counseling may be neither possible nor even preferable.[53-58] The practice, these authors maintain, may stand in tension with other professional obligations around informed consent, lead to decisions that are either objectively poor or do not optimally reflect patients' true preferences, and propagate implicit, discriminatory biases. Practitioners may hold differing understandings of what nondirective counseling means or how to engage in it. Perhaps most importantly, the relational bridges necessary for supporting individuals making sensitive, life-altering decisions may be impaired as providers conceal their authenticity behind a value-neutral "smokescreen."[54]

Given how deeply embedded the commitment to value neutrality is within prenatal counseling culture, communication training programs could be developed to enhance providers' comfort communicating about their values with patients. Thus far, an approach to more open and honest communication with patients about provider and institutional predilections has not been systematically attempted. We might find that sensitive engagement in such conversations creates genuine connections that enhance patients' decisions rather than undermine them. It might promote truly shared decision-making in which clinicians and providers mutually bear the moral burden of today's available technologies. Perhaps such a process would empower clinicians comfortably to answer questions such as "doctor, what would you do?" in a way that heightens patients' and clinicians' appreciation for each others' lived values. Hearing how clinicians articulate their deeply held values may help patients articulate their own.

Insofar as physician biases and institutional predilections may act similarly to financial conflicts of interest in unduly influencing the information, recommendations, and services offered to pregnant women when fetal conditions are diagnosed, tougher measures could also be considered to ameliorate their potential impact. More stringent criteria could be established to define what a "fetal care center" is and the services it should house. The AAP and ACOG recommend robust multidisciplinary oversight with in-house or referral mechanisms in place to support all potential decisions, including abortion.[47] Stronger steps would include mandating that (1) oversight be external, (2) control of centers with primary obstetrics services be separate and independent from pediatrics centers to which they may refer, and (3) obstetrics- and pediatrics-based centers that provide counseling in these circumstances be independent of any given insurance plan, particularly if the plan is selective regarding which services it will and will not cover and even more so if the insurance plan covers services selectively provided at its associated center.

Forceful measures like these may not be in many patients' best interests. Such strong processes may not all be necessary where more open and honest communication may suffice. Indeed, a compelling rationale exists for comprehensive, seamless healthcare delivery incorporating the obstetrics/pediatrics practice hybrid that Lucey imagined more than 50 years ago. The hope would be to create a counseling culture that permits legitimate variations in attitudes and practices to be discussed responsibly and that offers confidence in the due prioritization of reasonable patient preferences. At present, the only party facing any expectations for genuine transparency seems to be Crystal herself, and she needs help.

References

1. Lucey JF, Friedman E. Prospects in pediatrics: International conference on intrauterine fetal surgery. *Pediatrics.* 1965;35:813.
2. Liley AW. The use of amniocentesis and fetal transfusion in erythroblastosis fetalis. *Pediatrics.* 1965;35:836–47.
3. Casper M. *The Making of the Unborn Patient: A Social Anatomy of Fetal Surgery.* New Brunswick, NJ: Rutgers University Press; 1998.
4. Harrison MR. Fetal surgery: Trials, tribulations, and turf. *J Pediatr Surg.* 2003;38:275–82.
5. McMann CL, Carter BS, Lantos JD. Ethical issues in fetal diagnosis and treatment. *Am J Perinatol.* 2014;31:637–44.
6. Antiel RM. Ethical challenges in the new world of maternal-fetal surgery. *Semin Perinatol.* 2016;40:227–33.
7. Brown SD, Lyerly AD, Little MO. Lantos JD. Paediatrics-based fetal care: Unanswered ethical questions. *Acta Paediatrica.* 2008;97:1617–9.
8. Brown SD, Ecker JL, Ward JR, et al. Prenatally diagnosed fetal conditions in the age of fetal care: Does who counsels matter? *Am J Obstet Gynecol.* 2012;206:409 e1–11.
9. Kett JC, Woodrum DE, Diekema DS. A survey of fetal care centers in the United States. *J Neonatal Perinatal Med.* 2014;7:131–5.
10. Fost N, Chudwin D, Wikler D. The limited moral significance of "fetal viability." *Hastings Cent Rep.* 1980;10:10–3.
11. *Roe v. Wade,* 410 US 113, 93 SCt 705 (1973)

12. Peller AJ, Westgate MN, Holmes LB. Trends in congenital malformations, 1974–1999: Effect of prenatal diagnosis and elective termination. *Obstet Gynecol.* 2004;104:957–64.

13. Lyerly AD, Gates EA, Cefalo RC, Sugarman J. Toward the ethical evaluation and use of maternal-fetal surgery. *Obstet Gynecol.* 2001;98:689–97.

14. Devers PL, Cronister A, Ormond KE, Facio F, Brasington CK, Flodman P. Noninvasive prenatal testing/noninvasive prenatal diagnosis: The position of the National Society of Genetic Counselors. *J Genet Couns.* 2013;22:291–5.

15. Curlin FA, Lawrence RE, Chin MH, Lantos JD. Religion, conscience, and controversial clinical practices. *N Engl J Med.* 2007;356:593–600.

16. Antiel RM, Curlin FA, James KM, Tilburt JC. Physicians' beliefs and U.S. health care reform: A national survey. *N Engl J Med.* 2009;361:e23.

17. Yoon JD, Rasinski KA, Curlin FA. Moral controversy, directive counsel, and the doctor's role: Findings from a national survey of obstetrician-gynecologists. *Acad Med.* 2010;85:1475–81.

18. Combs MP, Antiel RM, Tilburt JC, Mueller PS, Curlin FA. Conscientious refusals to refer: Findings from a national physician survey. *J Med Ethics.* 2011;37:397–401.

19. Harris LH, Cooper A, Rasinski KA, Curlin FA, Lyerly AD. Obstetrician-gynecologists' objections to and willingness to help patients obtain an abortion. *Obstet Gynecol.* 2011;118:905–12.

20. Hersh ED, Goldenberg MN. Democratic and Republican physicians provide different care on politicized health issues. *Proc Natl Acad Sci USA.* 2016;113:11811–6.

21. Turner J, Preston L, Booth A, et al. What evidence is there for a relationship between organisational features and patient outcomes in congenital heart disease services? A rapid review. *Southampton (UK): NIHR Journals Library.* 2014 Nov. PMID: 25642567.

22. Kane JM, Canar J, Kalinowski V, Johnson TJ, Hoehn KS. Management options and outcomes for neonatal hypoplastic left heart syndrome in the early twenty-first century. *Pediatr Cardiol.* 2016;37:419–25.

23. Wernovsky G. The paradigm shift toward surgical intervention for neonates with hypoplastic left heart syndrome. *Arch Pediatr Adolesc Med.* 2008;162:849–54.

24. Prsa M, Holly CD, Carnevale FA, Justino H, Rohlicek CV. Attitudes and practices of cardiologists and surgeons who manage HLHS. *Pediatrics.* 2010;125:e625–30.

25. Kon AA, Prsa M, Rohlicek CV. Choices doctors would make if their infant had hypoplastic left heart syndrome: Comparison of survey data from 1999 and 2007. *Pediatr Cardiol.* 2013;34:348–53.

26. Spike JP. The ethics of treatment for hypoplastic left heart syndrome (HLHS). *Am J Bioeth.* 2017;17:65–6.

27. Kon AA, Ackerson L, Lo B. How pediatricians counsel parents when no "best-choice" management exists: Lessons to be learned from hypoplastic left heart syndrome. *Arch Pediatr Adolesc Med.* 2004;158:436–41.

28. Brown SD, Feudtner C, Truog RD. Prenatal decision-making for myelomeningocele: Can we minimize bias and variability? *Pediatrics.* 2015;136:409–11.

29. Adzick NS, Thom EA, Spong CY, et al. A randomized trial of prenatal versus postnatal repair of myelomeningocele. *N Engl J Med.* 2011;364:993–1004.

30. Moldenhauer JS. In utero repair of spina bifida. *Am J Perinatol.* 2014;31:595–604.

31. Johnson MP, Bennett KA, Rand L, et al. The Management of Myelomeningocele Study: Obstetrical outcomes and risk factors for obstetrical complications following prenatal surgery. *Am J Obstet Gynecol.* 2016;215:778 e1–e9.
32. Simpson JL. Fetal surgery for myelomeningocele: Promise, progress, and problems. *JAMA.* 1999;282:1873–4.
33. Bannister CM. The case for and against intrauterine surgery for myelomeningoceles. *Eur J Obstet Gynecol Reprod Biol.* 2000;92:109–13.
34. Grivell RM, Andersen C, Dodd JM. Prenatal versus postnatal repair procedures for spina bifida for improving infant and maternal outcomes. *Cochrane Database Syst Rev.* 2014:CD008825.
35. Antiel RM, Flake AW, Johnson MP, et al. Specialty-based variation in applying maternal-fetal surgery trial evidence. *Fetal Diagn Ther.* 2017;42:210–7.
36. Simpson JL, Greene MF. Fetal surgery for myelomeningocele? *N Engl J Med.* 2011;364:1076–7.
37. Adzick NS. Fetal surgery for myelomeningocele: Trials and tribulations. Isabella Forshall Lecture. *J Pediatr Surg.* 2012;47:273–81.
38. Meuli M, Moehrlen U. Fetal surgery for myelomeningocele is effective: A critical look at the whys. *Pediatr Surg Int.* 2014;30:689–97.
39. Antiel RM, Collura CA, Flake AW, et al. Physician views regarding the benefits and burdens of prenatal surgery for myelomeningocele. *J Perinatol.* 2017;37:994–8.
40. Shanmuganathan M, Sival DA, Eastwood KA, et al. Prenatal surgery for spina bifida: A therapeutic dilemma. Proceedings of the SHINE conference, Belfast. *Ir J Med Sci.* 2018;187:713–18.
41. Marteau T, Drake H, Bobrow M. Counselling following diagnosis of a fetal abnormality: The differing approaches of obstetricians, clinical geneticists, and genetic nurses. *J Med Genet.* 1994;31:864–7.
42. Brown SD, Donelan K, Martins Y, et al. Does professional orientation predict ethical sensitivities? Attitudes of paediatric and obstetric specialists toward fetuses, pregnant women and pregnancy termination. *J Med Ethics.* 2014;40:117–22.
43. Antiel RM, Curlin FA, Lantos JD, et al. Attitudes of paediatric and obstetric specialists towards prenatal surgery for lethal and non-lethal conditions. *J Med Ethics.* 2017.
44. Antiel RM, Flake AW, Collura CA, et al. Weighing the social and ethical considerations of maternal-fetal surgery. *Pediatrics.* 2017;140.
45. Kleinman A. The divided self, hidden values, and moral sensibility in medicine. *Lancet.* 2011;377:804–5.
46. Brown SD, Truog RD, Johnson JA, Ecker JL. Do differences in the AAP and ACOG positions on the ethics of maternal-fetal interventions reflect subtly divergent professional sensitivities to pregnant women and fetuses. *Pediatrics.* 2006;117:1382–7.
47. American College of Obstetricians and Gynecologists Committee on Ethics, American Academy of Pediatrics Committee on Bioethics, Committee opinion no. 501: Maternal-fetal intervention and fetal care centers. *Obstet Gynecol.* 2011;118:405–10.
48. Raju TN, Mercer BM, Burchfield DJ, Joseph GF, Jr. Periviable birth: Executive summary of a joint workshop by the Eunice Kennedy Shriver National Institute of Child Health and Human Development, Society for Maternal-Fetal Medicine, American Academy of Pediatrics, and American College of Obstetricians and Gynecologists. *Obstet Gynecol.* 2014;123:1083–96.

49. Goodman DC, Little GA. Data deficiency in an era of expanding neonatal intensive care unit care. *JAMA Pediatr.* 2018;172:11–2.
50. Thompson DF. Understanding financial conflicts of interest. *N Engl J Med.* 1993;329:573–76.
51. Kuppermann M, Pena S, Bishop JT, et al. Effect of enhanced information, values clarification, and removal of financial barriers on use of prenatal genetic testing: A randomized clinical trial. *JAMA.* 2014;312:1210–17.
52. Truog RD, Brown SD, Browning D, et al. Microethics: The ethics of everyday clinical practice. *Hastings Cent Rep.* 2015;45:11–17.
53. Clarke A. Is non-directive genetic counselling possible? *Lancet.* 1991;338:998–1001.
54. Williams C, Alderson P, Farsides B. Is nondirectiveness possible within the context of antenatal screening and testing? *Soc Sci Med.* 2002;54:339–47.
55. Reeder R, Veach PM, MacFarlane IM, LeRoy BS. Characterizing clinical genetic counselors' countertransference experiences: An exploratory study. *J Genet Couns.* 2017;26:934–47.
56. Clarke AJ, Wallgren-Pettersson C. Ethics in genetic counselling. *J Community Genet.* 2019;10:3–33.
57. Gould H, Hashmi SS, Wagner VF, Stoll K, Ostermaier K, Czerwinski J. Examining genetic counselors' implicit attitudes toward disability. *J Genet Couns.* 2019;28:1098–106.
58. Lowe C, Beach MC, Roter DL. Individuation and implicit racial bias in genetic counseling communication. *Patient Educ Couns.* 2020;103:804–10.

15

Ethical Issues in Academic Global Reproductive Health

Kayte Spector-Bagdady JD, MBE and Timothy R. B. Johnson MD, AM

Introduction

Since the 1980s, a clinical and research focus on "global reproductive health" has increased and commanded the attention of US medical schools and academic health centers.[1] This expansion is due to the increasing globalization of reproductive medicine and the clinicians-in-training who aspire to include global reproductive engagement in their professional careers. In fact, almost all US medical students have some type of global health training in their curriculum; almost 25% have at least one general "global health" experience prior to graduation.[2] But this increased interest has also generated new questions regarding best practices for global health engagement.

Two key global health issues have driven an increased interest in global *reproductive health* specifically. First, the HIV/AIDS epidemic, starting in the 1980s, was a powerhouse for change in understanding the globalization of disease. Beginning largely in communities of men who have sex with men, it quickly expanded among heterosexual women as well—with important implications for their own reproductive health and the health of their babies.[3] In response to the HIV/AIDS epidemic, US President George W. Bush's President's Emergency Plan for AIDS Relief (PEPFAR) worked in 60 countries to provide more than 11 million people with antiretroviral treatment. Since PEPFAR's initiation, almost 2 million babies have been born virus-free to HIV-positive women.[4] PEPFAR funds are also a major source of financial support for many centers for global health established at US universities— support which is then used to pay for clinical programs, training and education, and research purposes.

A second major catalyst for interest in global reproductive health was the 1985 landmark *Lancet* paper, "Maternal Mortality—A Neglected Tragedy.

Where Is the M in MCH?"[5] This paper highlighted for the world the high global burden of maternal mortality as well as the stark disparity between recent reductions in *infant* mortality as compared to steady or increasing instances of *maternal* mortality. This paper served to galvanize the international community and helped found the Safe Motherhood Initiative in 1987, to raise awareness of the devastating number of women dying in childbirth.[6,7] Resulting "Safe Motherhood" programs, less well-funded than those by PEPFAR, have focused on individual-level interventions (e.g., misoprostol and heat-stable oxytocin).

But while reproductive health is often approached from an individual clinical perspective, it also requires public health support resources such as access to diagnostic testing, a reliable method of drug distribution, and fulsome reproductive care systems. Thus the globalization of reproductive health has brought to light the more difficult challenges of capacity-building in affected communities.[8] Yet the topology of approaches of different global health experiences remains incredibly varied (Table 15.1).

The global health problems we have faced in the past, in combination with increasing student engagement and variable funding in the future, challenge us here to delve deeper into the ethical issues that must be considered for the development of efficient and effective US academic global reproductive health programs from the perspective of clinical care, education/training, and research.[9]

Academic Global Reproductive Health Programs

The first challenge of designing an academic reproductive health program is defining appropriate goals and approaches. Western bioethics has idealized

Table 15.1 Topology of global health experiences

Missionary work
Paid "service learning" trips
Professional exchanges
Surgical programs
Nongovernmental organizations
Medical "tourism" (e.g., student "white coat" adventures)
University-based programs

Table 15.2 Principles from the *Elmina Document on Human Resources for Health*

Trust	Mutual Respect
Communication	Accountability
Transparency	Leadership
Sustainability	

the principlist approach of assessing beneficence, nonmaleficence, autonomy, and justice in both clinical care and human subjects research.[10] But wholesale globalization of those principles is controversial because Western values are not universally shared or recognized. By forcing or expecting global communities to adopt Western standards one risks both "ethical imperialism"[11] as well as alienating critical partners. Building academic programs therefore requires bringing together the interests and priorities of both the host and international participants.

One example of such engagement is the *Elmina Document on Human Resources for Health*. This document reflects a Gates Foundation-funded exploration of fundamental principles underlying partnerships between institutions in high- and low-income countries.[12,13] These principles can assist in informing global reproductive health partnerships specifically (Table 15.2) with their focus on sustainability, accountability, and mutual respect.

As an example of these principles in context, many academic global health programs were established and are funded via PEPFAR. Thus are at risk of financial challenge when PEPFAR expires. But academic global health programs in high-income countries have a responsibility to maintain and not abandon these clinical, educational, and research services. Institutions that begin such engagement might have to prospectively commit other resources, tuition revenue, or reserves to maintain such critical global programmatic partnerships. Such structures, once established, often become co-dependent.

Clinical Global Reproductive Health Programs

A first area of global reproductive health engagement for consideration is clinical care programs. Two of the main models for such clinical programs are the *acute disease model* (often stemming from an infectious disease or a natural disaster) and the *primary care/capacity building model.* The acute disease model is based on epidemiologic principles of detection, medical treatment, and immunizations (when available). It is rooted in epidemic identification and invests resources in early detection, warning systems, and eradication.[14] The primary care/capacity building model, on the other hand, is particularly well-suited to clinical reproductive health programs because of its emphasis on holistic longitudinal care, such as family planning resources, and capacity building for trained attendance at delivery.

The recent Ebola outbreak in western Africa offers an excellent example of how a health campaign that was founded on the acute disease model failed to protect vulnerable populations when the needs of patients with Ebola intersected with the needs of pregnant women. As an example, in 2014, "the Ebola Fighters" were recognized by *Time Magazine* as "Persons of the Year."[15] One of the several cover photos for the issue featured Salome Karwah, a Liberian nursing assistant whose personal narrative exemplified a major success of the Ebola global health intervention. When she became ill with Ebola, she was admitted to her own hospital, where her father (a doctor), her mother, and many other of her family members had already died of Ebola. There she received specialized treatment—at huge cost compared to the health resources usually available in her country. This treatment was enabled in part by international global health players who responded to the Ebola epidemic, identified the major loci, treated those infected, limited its spread using advanced epidemiologic tools, and helped contain the disease (i.e., the acute disease model).[15]

But in 2016, Karwah was afflicted with a condition she would not survive: pregnancy. Days after delivery, she presented to her family hospital with what is easily recognizable to reproductive health professionals as eclampsia—pregnancy-associated seizures and hypertension. Unfortunately, her seizures and foaming mouth—in addition to her medical history as an Ebola survivor—frightened the staff. In addition, the drugs that should have been immediately available to treat eclampsia, both inexpensive and supposedly on every basic national formulary (magnesium sulfate and antihypertensive therapy), were not readily available to her. Thus, this Ebola survivor and hero died from stigma and a lack of access to a basic treatment for a common complication of pregnancy.[16]

The primary care/capacity building model therefore must also play a critical role in clinical health engagement in order to serve the needs of patients of reproductive age and pregnant patients specifically.[17-19] As Dr. Mahmoud

Fathalla of Egypt, former President of the International Federation of Gynecology and Obstetrics, eloquently stated: "Women are not dying because of untreatable diseases. They are dying because societies have yet to make the decision that their lives are worth saving."[20]

Global Reproductive Health Education and Training

A second common area of global reproductive health engagement is education and training. While growing, little is known about the impact of global reproductive health experiences for learners from high-income countries, although some literature is helpful to evaluating the impact of high-income training opportunities for learners from low-income countries.[21,22]

Throughout any such educational opportunity, it is critical to ensure that any potential benefits for students from high-income countries are balanced with care for patients and capacity building in low-income countries.[23] The pedagogical needs of these students must be secondary. Students should be prepared and trained *before* any such experiences as well. For example, it is not be appropriate for preclinical US medical students to travel to low-income countries and provide basic clinical care, such as blood pressure screening or physical exams. If students are not adequately trained or prepared to offer such services in the United States, they should not be providing them abroad. By the same token, if US institutions would not allow students from low-income countries of the same attainment level to perform such services on US patients, US students should not be allowed to do so abroad. This concept is critical to avoiding transforming medical pedagogy into "medical voyeurism."[24]

The type of services that students provide is critical. Preclinical students can benefit from an understanding of health education, basic disease, and epidemiology. Reproductive health education and healthy behavior education (e.g., regarding sexually transmitted diseases [STDs], HIV/AIDS prevention, human papilloma virus vaccination) can precede clinical experiences but are only appropriate for more senior students. Supervision under the rubric of competency and educational goals must be thoughtfully and consistently applied. Bilateral exchanges of students, where students from the hosting institution also are welcomed at the visiting institution, is also a necessary condition of global reproductive health partnerships. If students are not welcomed at each other's institutions equitably, it calls into question whether the relationship is actually a partnership or exploitative—where the gain is one-sided.[1,21,22,24]

Research

A third critical component of a robust global reproductive health partnerships is research, not only as a method of advancing faculty scholarship and student training, but also in terms of building infrastructure and attempting to address the health needs of the local community. Such a research partnership can help enable all of the goals of global reproductive health partnerships generally—engaging stakeholders, generating trust, and local capacity-building—but must be done not only with an eye to whether the work is getting done but also *how*.[12] While the ethical (and legal) issues relevant to international research are vast and already covered by the bioethics literature, global reproductive health research partnerships deserve a fresh look at how achieving the standard principles of Western research ethics programs can be enhanced by such a collaboration. From engaging the community, to conducting the research, to dissemination and publication of results, there are several areas of particular import to an effective and equitable global reproductive health research partnership.

Community Engagement

Setting a research agenda and structure must be a collaborative process in terms of defining goals from the students', institutions', and possibly the community's, perspectives. While "community-based participatory research" is a term of art intended to encompass research enabling community participation and control over a research process, there are also lessons to be learned from this formal collaborative process, with its emphasis on individual strengths[25] in a transcultural context. Applying community-based participatory research principles to international academic research collaborations allows for a model that respects a partner institution as a peer and representative of a unique community that exists "within larger social, political, and economic contexts."[26] For example, global reproductive health research collaborations should be built on partnership norms that include "mutual respect; recognition of the knowledge, expertise, and resource capacities of the participants in the process; and open communication."[26] In addition, research should be participatory, involve co-learning, and a focus on building local infrastructure and capacity—missions critical to reproductive healthcare generally.[25]

Broader than community-based participatory research principles, general "community engagement" is also critical for a collaborative approach to global reproductive health research in a transinstitutional and transcultural, context. Such community engagement can include a shared definition of research priorities, protocol design, and community consent via representative advisory boards.[27] This type of continuous engagement allows for "the integration of community norms, beliefs, customs, and cultural sensitivities" into the research enterprise.[28] Community engagement can represent a balance between culturally sensitive practices, such as requesting permission from a husband before asking consent from a pregnant research participant for an examination, while still ensuring a baseline of core human rights.[29] For example, the 2016 Council for International Organizations of Medical Science (CIOMS, an international nonprofit which provides ethical guidance on health research) Guidelines recommend "early and sustained" community engagement in the "design, development, implementation, design of the informed consent process and monitoring of research, and in the dissemination of its results."[27]

But a critical question for a global reproductive health research program then becomes, *who* is "the community"? In typical international research, the "community" (in contrast to the researchers), is the population from whom participants are derived. In global health research partnerships, the community is not only the research participants, but the partnering foreign institution: its administration, faculty, researchers, and students. In this case, researchers might or might not be part of the same community from which participants are derived. The goals of community engagement, demonstrating respect for traditions and norms as well as the successful conduct of research,[27] are the same in international research as in academic global partnerships—but academic global researchers must be cognizant of this additional layer of engagement with the partnering *academic institution*. They must ensure it is neither missed nor supplants robust engagement with the community of research participants.

Conducting the Research

Planning and approving a research protocol is not the only area of potential complication for global reproductive health research collaborations: there are also special considerations for researchers from high-income countries building such a program in low- and middle-income countries as "health in low-resource countries is often compromised by social determinants, such as poverty, malnutrition, poor education, unhealthy living conditions, and lack of access."[30] Three areas that particularly warrant attention include equitable subject section, research design, and ancillary care/research-related injury obligations.

A fundamental goal of research ethics is ensuring *equitable subject selection*, meaning that special protections are warranted for people placed in positions of vulnerability so that they are not exploited in research.[31] This goal is generally articulated to require that if research is going to be conducted with a population in a position of potential vulnerability (e.g., prisoners), then the protocol must be either specifically responsive to the health needs of that community or impractical to be carried out in another group.[31] As the US tome of research ethics, the *Belmont Report*, states

> selection of research subjects needs to be scrutinized in order to determine whether some classes are being systematically selected because of their easy availability, their compromised position, or their manipulability, rather than for reasons directly related to the problem being studied.[31]

For example, in the 1940s, US Public Health Service researchers went to Guatemala to test post-exposure prophylaxis STD regimens with commercial sex workers, prisoners, soldiers, and psychiatric patients. In addition to other fundamental issues, this research was not structured to benefit the vulnerable populations it utilized: instead, the goal of the research was to find an effective STD prophylaxis for inclusion in the US Army "pro kits." Such exploitation of these vulnerable international populations for the benefit of US citizens alone was highly unethical.[32,33]

By the same token, when populations in a position of potential vulnerability are used in reproductive health research, researchers should ensure specifically that there is thought put into post-trial accessibility of the successful research interventions for participants. For example, the 2002 international randomized controlled "Magpie Trial" demonstrated that magnesium sulfate halved the risk of eclampsia and "probably reduces the risk of maternal death" without significant negative effects.[34] But in at least several of the centers and countries that participated in the trial, magnesium sulfate was not available for routine clinical use for up to a decade after the study's publication (personal communication, on file with author TJ).

Another example was the Maternal-to-Child Transmission (MTCT) program focused on HIV/AIDS in Africa. This initiative provided antiretroviral therapy to pregnant women who were found to be HIV-positive after voluntary counseling and testing. HIV/AIDS-positive women were provided antiretroviral therapy for the duration of pregnancy, and the infants received neonatal antiretroviral therapy. The maternal-to-child transmission rate was reduced from 25% to less than 3%.[35] However, the initial MTCT programs did not generally provide for further antiretroviral therapy for participant mothers after delivery. Many eventually died from AIDS. Once this practice was highlighted to both donors and governments, the program name was changed to *Woman*-to-Child Transmission—with the recognition that the pregnant participants should continue to have post-delivery access to antiretroviral therapy both for their own sakes and for those of the children they had just borne.[36]

As these examples highlight, vulnerable participants should generally not be recruited to test an intervention they would have no reasonable way to access in the future.[31] In practice, this means ensuring that research proposed as part of global reproductive health research collaborations is tailored to specifically benefit the patients of the foreign institution or the community in which the research is being conducted, and thought must be put into post-trial accessibility of successful interventions as part of the proposal.

When designing protocols for global reproductive health research collaborations, special attention must also be paid to *trial design*. Research that tests an intervention against a placebo control when there is already a known safe and effective alternative available in the United States should be considered carefully. For example, in the 1990s, the antiretroviral drug zidovudine had been found to reduce HIV transmission by 67% when given to pregnant women during pregnancy and labor, and then to the infant postpartum.[37] However the US standard zidovudine protocol was unaffordable to many women in Asia and sub-Saharan Africa. Several studies were subsequently launched to identify a less costly dosage approach, but there was disagreement in the research ethics community regarding whether the modified zidovudine course should be compared to the "standard of care" in the participant community—which was nothing—or the established effective dosage available on the US market.[38]

While some international guidance recommends limiting the use of anything but the "best proven" intervention in a control arm (in the case of potential serious risk or irreversible harm of participants),[39] others have endorsed a middle ground that could be tailored to a particular community "given their health needs and the level of available medical and logistical infrastructure, cultural practices, genetics, and economic capacity to sustain treatment into the future."[28] It is critical for any global reproductive health research partnership to define ahead of time what "standard of care" for the control arm will be, taking into account both international ethics guidance as well as potential enhanced obligations generated by the unique collaboration of institutions.

A last area (for the purposes of this chapter) is potential ethical duties researchers might have by engaging in global reproductive health research collaborations in communities with inequitable or little access to healthcare. Two examples are responding to *research-related injury* or other *ancillary care obligations* for concomitant participant illness. Participants generally engage in research in return for little financial benefit and no guarantee of therapeutic effectiveness of the intervention. If participants become injured as a direct result of research, as opposed to because of normal progression of the illness at issue or other comorbidities, partnerships should seriously consider providing reparations and support for such participants so that they do not have to individually bear the costs of treatment for the injury.

Researchers should also question whether they might encounter other important health needs of their participants, particularly pregnant ones, during the conduct of their research—an ethical duty often called an "ancillary care obligation."[40] For example, do researchers focusing on midwifery-assisted birthing practices have the obligation to provide indicated antiretroviral treatment to participants in non-HIV/AIDS studies in developing countries? Global reproductive health research collaborations must weigh seriously potential ethical obligations to address other pressing health needs, particularly when their research is a unique vehicle for recognizing other illnesses (i.e., the disease is not otherwise readily apparent[40]) and the therapy is inexpensive, effective, and easy to deploy.

In all of these research ethics topics, global reproductive health research partnerships have a unique asset: the existing relationship between the institutions. Typically these critical ethical, scientific, and practical assessments as just discussed are made by the researchers and their approving institutional review board (IRB). However global reproductive health researchers should utilize this special relationship to not only request feedback on approach, but also to think creatively regarding deploying shared resources in the most effective and equitable fashion for both the international institutional and participant community.

In addition, issues already readily apparent in the US IRB structure may be compounded in an international one. For example, despite the limitations of attempting to internationalize Western conceptions of research ethics, local US IRBs are required to use them to approve protocols conducted under US federal regulations.[41] While liaising with the IRB at the local institution where the research will be conducted is of critical importance, that local IRB may feel pressured to "approve" research already so vetted in the United States.[42] This requirement for local IRB-approval of research might also tax already resource-poor institutions—if they even have one to begin with.[41]

In summary, the US study team must consider the following questions:

- Can the academic institutions work together such that post-trial access to an intervention can be sustained at the local institution after the protocol has come to a conclusion?
- Are the researchers sensitive to the effects of trial design on the participant community and, for example, recognize when building the protocol in a certain way might be coercive?
- Can global reproductive health researchers establish a partnership with local public health officials to recognize members of the participant community who may need better access to care or health education for future reproductive health infrastructure-building?

Dissemination and Publication

Global reproductive health research partnerships must also be cognizant of issues of dissemination and publication of their work.[12] For example, it is a good practice of community engagement that research results should be returned to the community (at the level revealed in publication).[27] This would likely not take the form of dissemination of peer-reviewed publications—which might be in a different language, at an inappropriate reading level, or too technical—but could be through summaries, discussions, or engagement with both the international academic and research participant community. As an example, it would be inappropriate for a global reproductive health research partnership to only offer the collaborating participants and institutional partners access to results behind a fee-for-service firewall.

This is not to say that publication in the peer-reviewed literature is not a critical component for successful academic global research collaborations[43] both in terms of the advancement of science as well as the careers of the local and international researchers. Researchers from the local institution should be engaged in all steps of the research—including design, approval, data collection, and analysis—but also in manuscript preparation and authorship of publications. For example, the *International Journal of Gynecology and Obstetrics* has a policy that local co-authors be included on papers from individual low- and middle-income countries to support "priorities for capacity building" as well as prevent the coopting of research by high-income countries.[44] Academic global research partnerships warrant particular scrutiny in ensuring equitable dissemination and publication at the conclusion of any research collaboration. Relatedly, data ownership, sharing, and future access and control should be codified in advance, with equally participating parties in the research having equitable access to the data moving forward.[45]

While none of these international research ethics issues regarding community engagement, conducting the research, and dissemination and publication is unique to global health research collaborations, an academic partnership is unique. As such, researchers must consider the best ways to leverage this relationship for the positive effect of the academic community, local community, and pregnant women with whom the work is intended to benefit.

Conclusion

Interest in and commitment to global reproductive health engagement has been increasing across the United States. US institutions—as well as their students, faculty, and staff—all have much to learn and share with global reproductive health partners. That said, all such engagements must be thoughtfully entered into, conducted, and exited. They should leave any low-income partners better off than they were before and certainly not any worse. Particularly in the areas of clinical care, training and education, and research in global reproductive health, there are particular standards against which we should hold and assess all of those involved. These standards are designed to enable fruitful pedagogy and collaboration and avoid medical voyeurism. All global engagements must represent a serious commitment not just from a center or a few affiliated colleagues, but also broadly from the institution, to commit to appropriate enabling and capacity building. We have much to learn from and in the area of global reproductive health engagement. It is only with thoughtful reflection and movement that we will actually accomplish what we set out to do.

References

1. Anderson FWJ, Wansom T. Beyond medical tourism: Authentic engagement in global health. *AMA J Eth VM* 2009;11(7):506–10.
2. Drain PK, Primack A, Hunt DD, et al. Global health in medical education: A call for more training and opportunities. *Acad Med.* 2007;82:226–30.
3. Chin J. Current and future dimensions of the HIV/AIDS pandemic in women and children. *Lancet.* 1990;336(8709):221–4.
4. PEPFAR. About us. 2017. https://www.pepfar.gov/about/270968.htm
5. Rosenfield A, Maine D. Maternal mortality: A neglected tragedy: Where is the M in MCH? *Lancet.* 1985;326(8446):83–5.
6. Thaddeus S, Maine D. Too far to walk: maternal mortality in context. *Newsl Womens Glob Netw Reprod Rights.* Jul–Sep 1991;(36):22–4.
7. Starrs AM. Safe motherhood initiative: 20 years and counting. *Lancet.* 2006;368(9542):1130–2.
8. Adetoro AA, Mani S, Abubakar A, et al. Capacity building of skilled birth attendants: A review of pre-service education curricula. *Midwifery.* 2013;29(7):e64–e72.
9. Kekulawala M, Johnson TRB. Ethical issues in global health engagement. *Semin Fetal Neonatal Med.* 2018;23:59–63.
10. Beauchamp TL, Childress JF. *Principles of Biomedical Ethics.* 7th ed. New York: Oxford University Press; 2012.
11. Macklin R. Unresolved issues in international research. *Kennedy Inst Ethics J.* 2001;11:17–36.
12. Anderson F, Donkor P, De Vries R, et al. Creating a charter of collaboration for international university partnerships: The Elmina Declaration for Human Resources for Health. *Acad Med.* 2014;89(8):1125–32.
13. Chattopadhyay S, De Vries R. Respect for cultural diversity in bioethics is an ethical imperative. *Med Health Care Philos.* 2013;16(4):639–45.
14. Padian NS, Holmes CB, McCoy SI, et al. Implementation science for the US President's Emergency Plan for AIDS Relief (PEPFAR). *J Acquir Immune Defic Syndr.* 2011;56(3):199–203.
15. Time. Person of the Year: The Ebola fighters. 2014 Dec 22–29.
16. Baker A. Liberian Ebola fighter, a Time person of the year, dies in childbirth. Time Health. 2017 Feb 27. http://time.com/4683873/ebola-fighter-time-person-of-the-year-salome-karwah/

17. Johnson CT, Johnson TRB, Adanu RMK. Obstetric surgery. In Debas H, Gawande A, Jamison D, Kruk M, eds. *Essential Surgery: Disease Control Priorities*. 3rd ed. Washington, DC: The International Bank for Reconstruction and Development/ World Bank; 2015 Apr 2: vol. 2, chap. 5, 77–94, PMID 26740991.

18. Mock CN, Donkor P, Gawande A, et al. Essential surgery: Key messages from Disease Control Priorities, 3rd edition. *Lancet*. 2015;385(9983):2209–19.

19. Anderson FWJ, Johnson TRB, DeVries R. Global health ethics: The case of maternal and neonatal survival. *Best Pract Res Clin Obstet Gynaecol*. 2017;43:125–35.

20. Fathalla MF. Human rights aspects of safe motherhood. *Best Pract Res Clin Obstet Gynaecol*. 2006;20:409–19.

21. Abedini NC, Danso-Bamfo S, Moyer CA, et al. Perceptions of Ghanaian medical students completing a clinical elective at the University of Michigan Medical School. *Acad Med*. 2014;89(7):1014–17.

22. Abendini NC, Danso-Bamfo S, Kolars JC, et al. Cross-cultural perspectives on the patient-provider relationship: A qualitative study exploring reflections from Ghanaian medical students following a clinical rotation in the United States. *BMC Med Educ*. 2015;15(161):doi 10.1186/s12909-015-0444-9.

23. Melby MK, Loh LC, Evert J, et al. Beyond medical "missions" to impact-driven Short-Term Experiences in Global Health (STEGHs): Ethical principles to optimize community benefit and learner experience. *Acad Med*. 2016;91(5):633–8.

24. Lawrence ER, Moyer C, Ashton C, Ibine BAR, Abedini NC, Spraggins Y, Kolars JC, Johnson TRB. Embedding international medical student electives within a 30-year partnership: The Ghana-Michigan collaboration. *BMC Med Educ*. 2020;20(1):189.

25. Minkler M. Ethical challenges for the "outside" researcher in community-based participatory research. *Health Educ Behav*. 2004;31(6):684–97.

26. Lance PM, Viruell-Fuentes E, Israel BA, et al. Can communities and academic work together on public health research? Evaluation results from a community-based participatory research partnership in Detroit. *J Urban Health*. 2001;78(3):495–507.

27. Council for International Organizations of Medical Sciences (CIOMS). *International Ethical Guidelines for Health-related Research Involving Humans*. 4th ed. Geneva: Author; 2016.

28. Presidential Commission for the Study of Bioethical Issues (PCSBI). *Moral Science: Protecting Participants in Human Subjects Research*. Washington, DC: Author; 2011.

29. Angell M. Ethical imperialism: Ethics in international collaborative clinical research. *N Engl J Med*. 1988;319(16):1081–3.

30. WHO. *Global Health Ethics Key Issues: Global Network of WHO Collaborating Centres for Bioethics*. Luxembourg: WHO; 2015.

31. National Commission for the Protection of Human Subjects of Biomedical and Behavioral Research (National Commission). *The Belmont Report: Ethical Principles and Guidelines for the Protection of Human Subjects Research*. 1979. Washington, DC: US Department of Health and Human Services; 1979.

32. Presidential Commission for the Study of Bioethical Issues (PCSBI). "Ethically impossible": STD research in Guatemala 1947 to 1948. Washington, DC: Author; 2010.

33. Spector-Bagdady K, Lombardo PA. US Public Health Service STD experiments in Guatemala (1946–1948) and their aftermath. *Ethics Hum Res*. 2019;41(2):29–34.

34. Magpie Trial Collaborative Group. Do women with pre-eclampsia, and their babies, benefit from magnesium sulphate? The Magpie Trial: A randomised placebo-controlled trial. *Lancet.* 2002;359(9321):1877–90.
35. Siegfried N, van der Merwe L, Brocklehurst P, et al. Antiretrovirals for reducing the risk of mother-to-child transmission of HIV infection. *Cochrane Database Syst Rev.* 2011;(7):CD003510.
36. Myer L, Rabkin M, Abrams EJ, et al. Focus on women: Linking HIV care and treatment with reproductive health services in the MTCT-Plus initiative. *Reprod Health Matters.* 2005;13(25):136–46.
37. Sperling RS, Shapiro DE, Coombs RW, et al. Maternal viral load, zidovudine treatment, and the risk of transmission of human immunodeficiency virus type 1 from mother to infant. *N Engl J Med.* 1996;335:1621–9.
38. Lurie P, Wolfe S. Unethical trials of interventions to reduce perinatal transmission of the human immunodeficiency virus in developing countries. *N Engl J Med.* 1997;337(12):853–6.
39. World Medical Association (WMA). Declaration of Helsinki: Ethical principles for medical research involving human subjects. 2013. http://www.wma.net/en/30publications/10policies/b3/
40. Richardson HS. *Moral Entanglements: The Ancillary-Care Obligations of Medical Researchers.* New York: Oxford University Press; 2012.
41. Alfano SL. Conducting research with human subjects in international settings: Ethical considerations. *Yale J Bio Med.* 2013;86(3):315–21.
42. London L. Ethical oversight of public health research: Can rules and IRBs make a difference in developing countries? *Am J Public Health.* 2002;92(7):1079–84.
43. Smith E, Hunt M, Master Z. Authorship ethics in global health research partnerships between researchers from low or middle income countries and high income countries. *BMC Medical Ethics.* 2014;15:42.
44. International Journal of Gynecology and Obstetrics (IJGO). Author guidelines. http://obgyn.onlinelibrary.wiley.com/hub/journal/10.1002/(ISSN)1879-3479/about/author-guidelines.html
45. Spector-Bagdady K. "The Google of Healthcare": Enabling the privatization of genetic bio/databanking. *Ann Epidemiol.* 2016;26(7):515–19.

Printed in the USA/Agawam, MA
June 23, 2021

776766.014